ESMO handbook
of principles of
translational research

ESMO handbook of principles of translational research

Edited by

Hakan Mellstedt
Stockholm, Sweden

Dirk Schrijvers
Antwerp, Belgium

Dimitrios Bafaloukos
Athens, Greece

Richard Greil
Innsbruck, Austria

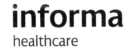

informa
healthcare

First published in the United Kingdom in 2007 by Informa Healthcare, 4 Park Square, Milton Park, Abingdon, Oxon OX14 4RN. Informa Healthcare is a trading division of Informa UK Ltd. Registered Office: 37/41 Mortimer Street, London W1T 3JH. Registered in England and Wales Number 1072954.

Tel.: +44 (0)20 7017 6000
Fax.: +44 (0)20 7017 6699
E-mail: info.medicine@tandf.co.uk
Website: www.informahealthcare.com

A CIP record for this book is available from the British Library.
Library of Congress Cataloging-in-Publication Data

Data available on application

ISBN 10: 0 415 394325
ISBN 13: 978 0 415 39432 1

Distributed in North and South America by
Taylor & Francis
6000 Broken Sound Parkway, NW (Suite 300)
Boca Raton, FL 33487, USA

Within Continental USA
Tel: 1(800)272 7737; Fax: 1(800)374 3401
Outside Continental USA
Tel: (561)994 0555; Fax: (561)361 6018
E-mail: orders@crcpress.com

Distributed in the rest of the world by
Thomson Publishing Services
Cheriton House
North Way
Andover, Hampshire SP10 5BE, UK
Tel.: +44 (0)1264 332424
E-mail: tps.tandfsalesorder@thomson.com

Composition by C&M Digitals (P) Ltd, Chennai, India
Printed and bound in Italy by Printer Trento

Contents

Foreword

This ESMO Handbook of Principles of Translational Research is an important new addition to the ESMO Handbook series that have been so well received by the oncology community. Translational research is a broad field that is focused on accelerating the transfer of knowledge from the laboratory to the patient and back. In recent years we have already witnessed some impressive benefits from this approach such as the emergence of novel targeted therapies, identification of gene mutations and expression profiles predictive of tumor behavior and response to therapy and advances in tumor immunology and angiogenesis, just to name a few. This Handbook is aimed at further facilitating the understanding of the key important areas of translational research and is directed to a general oncology audience as well as to those involved in research. The three distinguished editors of this Handbook, Drs Greil, Mellstedt and Schrijvers have done a superb job at identifying the key topics in the field and have incorporated superb contributors. All important areas of translational research are being covered from the basic mechanisms governing the malignant cell to new targets, gene and protein profiling and drug development issues. I am confident that you will find this book to be an enjoyable and useful companion in your daily work.

– José Baselga
ESMO President-Elect

Principles of normal cell biology

A Vandebroek, D Schrijvers
Ziekenhuisnetwerk Antwerpen–Middelheim,
Antwerp, Belgium

Normal cell structure

Introduction

Cells are the basic units of the human body. Nearly all types of cells have essentially the same internal structure. Most cells contain cytoplasm, cell organelles, a nucleus, and other structures contained by a plasma membrane (Figure 1.1).

▨ The cytoplasm is the viscous content, including proteins, cell organelles, metabolites and ions.
▨ Cell organelles are membrane-bound structures such as mitochondria, the endoplasmic reticulum, the Golgi apparatus, and lysosomes.
▨ The nucleus has an envelope and contains nucleoplasm, deoxyribonucleic acid (DNA) organized as chromosomes, and the nucleolus, where ribosomes are constructed.
▨ Other structures in the cytoplasm are proteasomes, centrioles, ribosomes, the cytoskeleton, and various proteins and small molecules.
▨ The plasma membrane is the membrane surrounding the cytoplasm, and consists of a phospholipid bilayer and associated proteins and carbohydrates.

Cell organelles and structures

Mitochondria

A cell contains many mitochondria, which consist of two membranes and contain their own mitochondrial DNA (mtDNA) encoding for some mitochondrial proteins and ribonucleic acid (RNA). However, most proteins that function in mitochondria are encoded by nuclear DNA.

The function of mitochondria is to produce adenosine triphosphate (ATP), which carries energy to power most cellular processes.

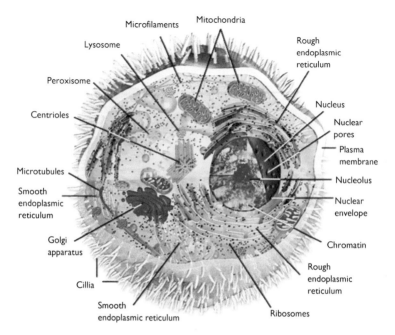

Figure 1.1 Cell structure

Endoplasmic reticulum

The endoplasmic reticulum (ER) can be divided into rough and smooth ER. The function of the rough ER is to process newly ribosome-synthesized peptides and its surface is usually associated with ribosomes, while the smooth ER is involved in the synthesis and metabolism of lipids.

Golgi apparatus

The Golgi apparatus is the major site for sorting and modification of proteins and lipids. After proteins have been sorted at the rough ER, they are enclosed in transport vesicles and carried to the Golgi apparatus. Some proteins are modified into glycoproteins and then transported to other destinations.

Lysosomes

The function of lysosomes is to degrade various macromolecules in the cell. They contain nucleases for degrading DNA and RNA, proteases for degrading proteins, and other enzymes for degrading polysaccharides and lipids.

Proteasome

The proteasome is a large, cylindrical, multisubunit protein complex, which is present in high amounts in both cytoplasm and nucleus. Its function is the elimination of cellular proteins, including those that have been tagged for degradation by polyubiquitination. Proteins entering the proteasome are stripped of their ubiquitin, unfolded, and subsequently degraded through catalytic activities within the core of the proteasome. Protein substrates enter this proteasome core through the outer ring of the proteasome if they are unfolded. A complex located at the end of the proteasome core catalyzes the unfolding of proteins and their transport into the central chamber, where proteolytic sites located on subunits in the inner rings cleave the proteins.

Centrioles

Centrioles are short cylindrical organelles, found in pairs arranged at right-angles to each other at the microtubule organizing center (MTOC) or centrosome.

Centrosomes

Centrosomes are composed of two orthogonally arranged centrioles surrounded by an amorphous mass of pericentriolar material. The centrosome organizes formation of a spindle during mitosis or meiosis, and is involved in the cell cycle progression.

Ribosomes

Ribosomes are organelles composed of ribosomal RNA (rRNA) and ribosomal proteins. They translate messenger RNA (mRNA) into proteins. Ribosomes can float freely in the cytoplasm or bind to the ER and the nuclear envelope.

Nucleosome

DNA is packaged into a compact structure by specialized proteins known as histones. The complex of DNA plus histones is called chromatin. The nucleosome is a subunit of chromatin composed of a short length of DNA wrapped around a core of histone proteins.

Nucleolus

The nucleolus is part of the nucleus. Its main function is the production and assembly of ribosome components. It is made of proteins and rDNA.

Cell cycle

Cell cycle phases

Most cells do not divide, and remain in interphase (G_0). After stimulation by internal or external signals, a cell can enter the cell cycle. The cell cycle is the process by which a cell divides, and is a sequence of growth ('gap 1': G_1), DNA synthesis (S), growth ('gap 2': G_2), and cell division or mitosis (M) phases.

G_1 phase

During G_1 phase, the cell acquires ATP and increases in size.

S phase

During S phase, replication of the original DNA, resulting in two identical copies, occurs. DNA is composed of nucleotides, each consisting of a nitrogenous base (cytosine, thymine, adenine, or guanine), deoxyribose (a sugar), and a phosphate group. It is organized in a double helix with complementary strands held together by hydrogen bonding between the bases: adenine pairs with thymine, and cytosine pairs with guanine. DNA replication involves many nucleotides, enzymes, and energy.

- DNA polymerases unzip the helix by breaking hydrogen bonds between bases. Once the polymerases have opened the helix, a replication fork forms. New nucleotides are placed in the fork and link to the corresponding parent nucleotide. Normal replication of a linear DNA strand by DNA polymerase is initiated from the site of a bound primer, and can proceed only from a 5′ position to a 3′ position. Since no primer is bound at the extreme 5′ end of each chromosome, there is a gap in replication, leading to a progressive shortening of daughter strands with each round of DNA replication.
- At the end of each DNA strand, there are a few hundred to a thousand similar sequences of six nucleotides (thymidine, thymidine, adenosine, guanosine, guanosine, guanosine: TTAGGG). These are called telomeres, and

their function is to maintain chromosomal integrity. They are synthesized by telomerase, a ribonucleoprotein enzyme composed of both RNA and protein. The RNA component contains nucleotides that are complementary to those present in the telomere. By reverse transcription, telomerase makes a DNA copy of its own RNA sequence, which is then fused to the 3′ terminus of the chromosome. The extension of telomeres by telomerase is required to counter the normal shrinkage of chromosomes that occurs after each round of DNA replication.

■ The breaks in DNA strands are repaired by topoisomerases I and II.

G_2 phase

During G_2 phase, the cell undergoes a second phase of growth and energy acquisition.

M phase

Mitosis is the process of forming identical daughter cells by replicating and dividing the original chromosomes. The condensed replicated chromosomes consist of two molecules of DNA and their associated histone proteins, known as chromatids. The area where both chromatids are in contact with each other is the centromere and is the point where the spindle apparatus attaches.

■ During prophase, chromatin condenses, the nuclear envelope dissolves, centrioles divide and migrate, microtubules form, and the spindle forms.
■ During metaphase, chromosomes migrate to the equator of the spindle, where the spindles attach to the centromere.
■ During anaphase, separation of the centromeres begins and the chromosomes are pulled to opposite poles of the spindle.
■ During telophase, chromosomes reach the poles of their respective spindles, the nuclear envelope reforms, chromosomes uncoil into chromatin, and the nucleolus reforms.

Cell cycle regulation

Cell cycle progression is regulated by surveillance mechanisms or cell cycle checkpoints, which ensure the ordered execution of cell cycle events.

Cell cycle progression is driven by a number of cyclin-dependent kinases (CDKs) that are activated by specific regulatory proteins (cyclins). There are corresponding cell cycle inhibitory proteins (CDK inhibitors: CDKIs) that serve as negative regulators of the cell cycle and stop the cell from proceeding to the next phase of the cycle.

G_1/S cell cycle checkpoint

The G_1/S cell cycle checkpoint controls the passage from the first 'gap' phase (G_1) into the DNA synthesis phase (S). Two cell cycle kinases (CDK4/6–cyclin D and CDK2–cyclin E) and the transcription complex of the retinoblastoma tumor suppressor gene product (pRb) and E2F regulate the G_1/S cell cycle checkpoint.

■ In its active state, pRb forms an inhibitory complex with a group of transcription factors, E2F–DP, each of which is a heterodimer of an E2F protein (E2F-1, -2, and -3) and a DP protein (Dp-1, -2, -3). The activity of pRb is modulated by sequential phosphorylation by CDK4/6–cyclin D and CDK2–cyclin E. When pRb is partially phosphorylated by the CDK4/6–CDKs, it remains bound to E2F–DP. This transcription factor is still able to transcribe some genes such as *CCNE*, encoding cyclin E. Cyclin E then binds to CDK2 and this active complex then completely hyperphosphorylates pRb, thus releasing the E2F–DP heterodimer and fully activating the E2F transcription factors. This results in transcriptional activation of S-phase proteins.
■ In addition to pRb, CDK2 phosphorylates other substrates involved in DNA replication.

S-phase progression

■ Early in S phase, cyclins D and E are targeted by ubiquitination for proteasome degradation.
■ The production of cyclin A and its complexing with CDK2 enables S-phase progression, with the production of other enzymes and proteins involved in DNA synthesis.
■ Orderly S-phase progression requires the timely inactivation of E2F, in part accomplished by cyclin A-dependent kinase activity. CDK2–cyclin A stably associates with E2F-1 and directs phosphorylation of the E2F–DP heterodimer, neutralizing its DNA-binding capacity.
■ During late S and throughout G_2, cells prepare for mitosis by increasing levels of cyclins A and B. As the level of cyclin B rises, it forms a complex with cdc2 (CDK1) in the cytoplasm, where it remains until mitosis, at which point it shuttles into the nucleus.

G_2/M cell cycle checkpoint

The G_2/M cell cycle checkpoint prevents the cell from entering mitosis if the genome is damaged. It is regulated by cdc2–cyclin B kinase.

- During G_2 phase, cdc2 is maintained in an inactive state by the kinases Wee1 and Myt1.
- Cdc25 is a protein phosphatase responsible for dephosphorylating and activating cdc2. Cdc25 is phosphorylated throughout interphase but not in mitosis.

M-phase progression

Progression through mitosis is dependent on the anaphase-promoting complex (APC)/cyclosome and the degradation of cyclin B.

During mitosis, the assembly of a bipolar spindle by the centrosome is essential for preservation of genetic fidelity between daughter cells. The assembly is monitored by a checkpoint that senses microtubule defects or aberrant kinetochore attachment.

Survivin is implicated in the regulation of the mitotic spindle and in the preservation of cell viability, due to its expression during cell division in a cell cycle-dependent manner and its localization to the mitotic apparatus; cyclin B1/cdc2 activity during mitosis plays a critical role in survivin expression and function in cell viability.

Centrosome maturation

Centrosome maturation is critical for cell division and is regulated by several kinases, including Polo kinase and Aurora kinase.

- Centrosome maturation begins with centriole duplication, which occurs in G_1 and is triggered by CDK2–cyclin E and CDK2–cyclin D activity.
- Elongation of the centriole occurs throughout S phase, so that, by prophase, the cell has two pairs of centrioles within the pericentriolar material.
- Polo kinase is involved in recruiting tubulin and in activating the ASP ('abnormal spindles gene product') protein.
- Aurora kinase is also involved in centrosome maturation. It is required for correct spindle pole structure and bipolarity of the spindle, and appears to be essential in the duplication/separation stage of the centriole cycle.

p53

p53 (encoded by the *TP53* gene) is a transcription factor regulated by phosphorylation. p53 inhibits the cell from progressing through the cell cycle if there is damage to the DNA. It stops the cell at a checkpoint until repairs can be made, or causes apoptosis if the damage cannot be repaired.

Protein metabolism

DNA transcription and translation

Transcription

Every gene on a chromosome encodes a polypeptide. DNA is translated into polypeptides by transcription of a DNA template into RNA, with the RNA code being translated into an amino acid sequence – a protein.

During interphase, RNA polymerase opens the DNA double strand, and only one strand of DNA is transcribed, starting at a promotor region, from RNA nucleotides available in the chromatin. There are three different RNA polymerases:

- RNA polymerase I synthesizes rRNA.
- RNA polymerase II synthesizes mRNA and some small nuclear RNA (snRNA) involved in RNA splicing.
- RNA polymerase III synthesizes rRNA and transfer RNA (tRNA).

mRNA genes have a basic structure consisting of coding exons and non-coding introns, two types of basal promoters, and a number of different transcriptional regulatory domains. The basal promoter elements are named CCAAT boxes and TATA boxes. The TATA box resides 20–30 bases upstream of the transcriptional starting site. Numerous proteins ('transcription factors regulating RNA polymerase II': TFIIA) interact with the TATA box. The CCAAT box resides 50–130 bases upstream of the transcriptional starting site, and a protein known as C/EBP ('CCAAT-box/enhancer-binding protein') binds to the CCAAT-box element.

There are many other regulatory sequences in mRNA genes that bind various transcription factors. The number and type of regulatory elements vary with each mRNA gene. Different combinations of transcription factors can also exert differential regulatory effects upon transcriptional initiation. Various cell types express characteristic combinations of transcription factors, and this is the major mechanism for cell-type specificity in the regulation of mRNA gene expression.

The most common recognition pattern between transcription factors and DNA is an interaction between an α-helical domain of the factor and about five base-pairs within the major groove of the DNA helix. There are hundreds of transcription factor classes with specific DNA-binding domains. They are often classified according to the type of DNA-binding domain they contain, and include, among others:

- Steroid receptors (e.g., glucocorticoid receptors, thyroid hormone receptors, and retinoic acid receptors) are activated by binding to a particular steroid.
- Zinc-finger proteins have regions that fold around a central zinc ion, producing a compact domain from a relatively short length of the polypeptide chain.
- Leucine zipper proteins have a leucine residue in every seventh position. A leucine zipper in one polypeptide interacts with a zipper in another polypeptide to form a dimer.

Interaction of activated transcription factors with DNA and RNA polymerase allows transcription of specific DNA sequences to mRNA.

Ligand (e.g., hormone) binding to a nuclear heterodimeric receptor located in the nucleus regulates its activity as a transcription factor. When nuclear receptors are bound to their cognate sites in DNA, they act as repressors or activators of transcription, depending on whether the ligand occupies the ligand-binding site.

- In the absence of a ligand, these nuclear receptors direct histone deacetylation at nearby nucleosomes.
- In the presence of a ligand, the ligand-binding domain undergoes a conformational change and can directly hyperacetylate histones in nearby nucleosomes, thereby reversing the repressing effects of the free ligand-binding domain. The N-terminal activation domain in these receptors then interacts with additional factors, stimulating the cooperative assembly of an initiation complex.

Homodimeric receptors are found in both the cytoplasm and the nucleus. Their activity is regulated by controlling their transport from the cytoplasm to the nucleus. In the absence of hormones, the receptor is anchored in the cytoplasm as a large protein aggregate complexed with inhibitor proteins (e.g., heat-shock protein (Hsp)90), the receptor cannot interact with target genes, and so no transcriptional activation occurs. Hormone binding releases the receptor from its cytoplasmatic anchor, allowing it to enter the nucleus, where it can bind to response elements associated with target genes, activating transcription by directing histone hyperacetylation and facilitating cooperative assembly of an initiation complex.

Translation

Translation is the process of converting mRNA into an amino acid sequence. mRNA consists of a sequence of codons (one codon is made up by three bases). A codon may encode one of the 20 essential amino acids. There are 61 amino acid coding codons and 3 termination codons, which stop the process of translation.

mRNA is transported out of the nucleus to ribosomes. The smaller subunit of a ribosome has a binding place for mRNA, while the larger subunit has two binding sites for tRNA. tRNA consists of an anticodon (three bases), which is the complement of a codon, and an amino acid. The amino acid linkage is controlled by amino-acyl–tRNA synthetases.

After an initiation phase, the amino acids form a strand during the elongation phase. When a termination codon is encountered, a releasing factor binds to the ribosomal site, and translation halts.

Protein modification and repair

After translation, chaperone proteins assist the amino acid strand or polypeptide to attain a functional conformation as a new protein and guide the polypeptide at the site in the cell where it carries out its functions.

Stress to the cell causes protein denaturation, with the protein unfolding and becoming denatured and insoluble. The denatured proteins tend to stick to each other, precipitate, and form inclusion bodies.

The chaperone machine, consisting of three proteins (Hsp70, Hsp40 and nucleotide-exchange factor) can repair unfolded proteins. Hsp70 binds to a damaged polypeptide, assisting it to fold correctly and thus regain its native conformation. Distinctive functional domains in a chaperone molecule recognize a polypeptide in need of assistance, interact with another chaperone to build a chaperoning complex, and network with other chaperoning complexes or with a protein-degrading machine such as the ubiquitin–proteasome system.

Regulation of protein production

Production of proteins is controlled at different levels:

■ Transcriptional control – when and how often a gene is transcribed.
■ Gene regulatory proteins (co-activators and co-suppressors) can act even when they are bound to DNA thousands of nucleotide pairs away from the promoter that they influence. This means that a single promoter can be controlled by an almost unlimited number of regulatory sequences scattered along the DNA.

- RNA polymerase II, which transcribes all protein-encoding genes, cannot initiate transcription on its own. It requires a set of proteins (general transcription factors), which must be assembled at the promoter before transcription can start. This assembly process provides multiple steps at which the rate of transcription initiation can be speeded up or slowed down in response to regulatory signals.
- The packaging of DNA into chromatin through histone modifications and nucleosome remodeling provides opportunities for regulation.
- RNA processing control – how the RNA transcript is spliced or otherwise processed.
- RNA transport and localization control – selecting which completed mRNAs in the cell nucleus are exported to the cytosol and determining where in the cytosol they are localized.
- Translational control – which mRNAs in the cytoplasm are translated by ribosomes.
- mRNA degradation control – selectively destabilizing certain mRNA molecules in the cytoplasm.
- Protein activity control – selectively activating, inactivating, degrading, or compartmentalizing specific protein molecules after they have been made.

Protein degradation

The proteolytic machinery of cells is highly selective and tightly regulated, since the accelerated destruction of essential proteins or the failure to degrade a short-lived regulatory protein may change cell function:

- Rapid removal of rate-limiting enzymes and regulatory proteins is essential for the control of growth and metabolism.
- Rapid degradation of specific proteins permits adaptation to new physiological conditions.
- The degradation rate of specific proteins may change dramatically under different conditions.
- Protein breakdown provides quality control by selectively eliminating abnormally folded proteins that have arisen through mutations, biosynthetic errors, or oxygen free-radical damage.

Mechanisms

Lysosomes

Lysosomes are membrane-bound vesicles that contain several acid proteases and other hydrolases.

- Extracellular proteins undergo endocytosis and are completely degraded within lysosomes. This endosome–lysosome proteolytic pathway may also generate peptides that are presented to the immune system on cell surface major histocompatibility complex (MHC) class II molecules and elicit antibody or inflammatory responses.
- Cell membrane proteins may also be degraded within lysosomes (e.g., downregulation of receptors). After ligands bind to membrane receptors, the rate of endocytosis and degradation in lysosomes is accelerated.
- Some cytosolic proteins are degraded by engulfment in autophagic vacuoles that fuse with lysosomes.

Lysosomal proteolysis is not quantitatively important in the normal turnover of most cellular proteins.

Ubiquitin–proteasome

The ubiquitin–proteasome pathway degrades most cellular proteins by a multienzymatic energy-dependent process.

- Proteins are first marked for degradation by covalent linkage to the small protein cofactor ubiquitin. The carboxyl end of ubiquitin is first activated through conversion to a thiol ester by an ATP-requiring enzyme, E1. Activated ubiquitin is then transferred by E1 to one of a family of carrier proteins called E2 proteins, and the carboxyl group of ubiquitin is coupled by a ubiquitin–protein ligase (E3) to the amino groups of lysines in the protein substrate.
- The ubiquitin-conjugation reactions are repeated, forming a chain of five or more ubiquitins linked to each other and then to the protein substrate.
- Modification of the protein leads to its rapid degradation by the proteasome, which requires ATP to function. The proteins are cut progressively into small peptides of 6–12 amino acids until they are completely degraded. These peptides are released and rapidly hydrolyzed to amino acids by cytosolic exopeptidases, except for the peptides transported to the cell surface by MHC class I molecules.

Signal transduction

Signal transduction at the cellular level refers to signaling from outside the cell to the inside or within the cell, via:

- Movement of ions either into or out of the cell through ion channels after ligand binding. These ion movements result in changes in the electrical potential of the cells that, in turn, propagate the signal through the cell.

- Coupling of ligand–receptor interactions to intracellular events such as phosphorylation by tyrosine kinases and/or serine/threonine kinases. Protein phosphorylation changes enzyme activity and protein conformation. The eventual outcome is an alteration in cellular activity and changes in gene expression.

Classifications of signal-transducing receptors

There are three major classes of signal-transducing receptors:

- Receptors that penetrate the plasma membrane (extracellular, transmembrane, and intracellular domain) and have intrinsic enzymatic activity, such as:
    - tyrosine kinases: e.g., platelet-derived growth factor (PDGF), epidermal growth factor (EGF), and fibroblast growth factor (FGF) receptors
    - tyrosine phosphatases: e.g., CD45 protein of T cells and macrophages
    - guanylate cyclases: e.g., natriuretic peptide receptors
    - serine/threonine kinases: e.g., activin and transforming growth factor (TGF) receptors

Receptors with intrinsic tyrosine kinase activity are capable of autophosphorylation as well as phosphorylation of other substrates. Several families of receptors lack intrinsic enzymatic activity, but are coupled to intracellular tyrosine kinases by direct protein–protein interactions.

- Receptors that are coupled, inside the cell, to guanosine triphosphate (GTP)-binding and hydrolyzing proteins (G-proteins). Receptors that interact with G-proteins all have a structure characterized by seven transmembrane spanning domains. These receptors are termed serpentine receptors (e.g., adrenergic receptors, hormone receptors for glucagon, angiotensin, vasopressin, and bradykinin).
- Intracellular receptors that upon ligand binding migrate to the nucleus where the ligand–receptor complex directly affects gene transcription.

Receptor tyrosine kinases

Receptor tyrosine kinases (RTKs) generally have a structure comprising four major domains:

- an extracellular ligand-binding domain
- an intracellular tyrosine kinase domain
- an intracellular regulatory domain
- a transmembrane domain

Table 1.1 Characteristics of common classes of receptor tyrosine kinases

Class	Structural features of class	Examples
I	Cysteine-rich sequences	Epidermal growth factor receptor (EGFR, HER1), HER2/*neu* (c-ErbB2) HER3 (c-ErbB3)
II	Cysteine-rich sequences; characterized by disulfide-linked heterotetramers	Insulin receptor, insulin-like growth factor I receptor (IGF-IR)
III	Contain five immunoglobulin-like domains as well as the kinase domain	Platelet-derived growth factor receptors (PDGFR A and B), c-Kit (stem cell factor receptor, SCFR)
IV	Contain three immunoglobulin-like domains as well as the kinase domain; acidic domain	Fibroblast growth factor receptors (FGFR1, 2, 3, 4)
V	Contain seven immunoglobulin-like domains as well as the kinase domain	Vascular endothelial growth factor receptor (VEGFR)
VI	Heterodimeric like the class II receptors, except that one of the two protein subunits is completely extracellular. HGFR is the product of a proto-oncogene originally identified as the MET oncogene	Hepatocyte growth factor receptor (HGFR, Met), scatter factor receptor
VII	Contain no or few cysteine-rich domains; NGFR (TrkA) has a leucine-rich domain	Neurotrophin receptor family: TrkA (nerve growth factor receptor, NGFR), TrkB, TrkC

TrK: Tyrosine kinase

RTK proteins are classified into families based upon structural features in their extracellular portions, which include cysteine-rich domains, immunoglobulin-like domains, leucine-rich domains, Kringle domains, cadherin domains, fibronectin type III repeats, discoidin I-like domains, acidic domains, and EGF-like domains (Table 1.1).

Many receptors that have intrinsic tyrosine kinase activity, as well as the tyrosine kinases that are associated with cell surface receptors, contain tyrosines residue that upon phosphorylation interact with other proteins of the signaling cascade. These other proteins contain a domain of amino acid sequences that is termed the SH2 domain ('Src homology domain 2'). Another protein–protein interaction domain identified in many signal transduction proteins is related to a third domain in Src (the product of the proto-oncogene *SRC*), identified as the SH3 domain.

The interactions of SH2-domain-containing proteins with RTKs or receptor-associated tyrosine kinases lead to tyrosine phosphorylation of the SH2-containing proteins. The result of phosphorylation of SH2-containing proteins that have enzymatic activity is an alteration in activity. Several SH2-containing proteins that have intrinsic enzymatic activity include phospholipase C (PLC), the proto-oncogene *RAS*-associated GTPase-activating protein (Ras-GAP), phosphatidylinositol 3'-kinase (PI3-K), protein phosphatase-1C (PTP1C), as well as members of the Src family of protein tyrosine kinases.

Non-receptor protein tyrosine kinases

There are numerous intracellular protein tyrosine kinases (PTKs) that are responsible for phosphorylation of intracellular proteins on tyrosine residues following activation of cellular growth and proliferation signals.

Two distinct families of non-receptor PTKs are now recognized:

- The archetypal PTK family related to the Src protein.
- A second family related to the Janus kinases (Jaks).

Most of the proteins of both families of non-receptor PTKs couple to cellular receptors that lack enzymatic activity themselves. This class of receptors includes all of the cytokine receptors (e.g., the interleukin-2 (IL-2) receptor) as well as the CD4 and CD8 cell surface glycoproteins of T cells and the T-cell antigen receptor (TCR).

The insulin receptor (IR) is another example of receptor signaling through protein interaction. This receptor has intrinsic tyrosine kinase activity, but does not directly interact, following autophosphorylation, with enzymatically active proteins containing SH2 domains (e.g. PI3-K or PLC). Instead, the principal IR substrate is a protein termed IRS-1. IRS-1 contains several motifs that resemble SH2-binding consensus sites for the catalytically active subunit of PI3-K. These domains allow complexes to form between IRS-1 and PI3-K.

15

Receptor serine/threonine kinases

The receptors for the TGF-α superfamily of ligands have intrinsic serine/threonine kinase (RSTK) activity. There are more than 30 multifunctional proteins of the TGF-α superfamily, which also includes the activins, inhibins, and bone morphogenetic proteins (BMPs). This superfamily of proteins can induce and/or inhibit cellular proliferation or differentiation, and regulate migration and adhesion of various cell types.

Another effect of TGF-α is regulation of progression through the cell cycle. One nuclear protein involved in the responses of cells to TGF-α is the proto-oncogene product c-Myc.

Non-receptor serine/threonine kinases

There are several serine/threonine kinases that function in signal transduction pathways. The two more commonly known are cyclic adenosine monophosphate (cAMP)-dependent protein kinase (PKA) and protein kinase C (PKC). Additional serine/threonine kinases important for signal transduction are the mitogen-activated protein kinases (MAP kinases).

- The PKC family comprises at least ten proteins. Each of these enzymes exhibits specific patterns of tissue expression and activation by lipid and calcium. PKCs are involved in the signal transduction pathways initiated by certain hormones, growth factors, and neurotransmitters. Phosphorylation of various proteins by PKCs can lead to either increased or decreased activity. One important activity of PKCs is phosphorylation of the EGF receptor (EGFR), which downregulates the tyrosine kinase activity of the receptor. This limits the length of the cellular responses initiated through EGFR.
- MAP kinases (also known as extracellular-signal regulated kinases, ERKs) are classified based on their in vitro substrates:
  - microtubule-associated protein-2 kinase (MAP2 kinase)
  - myelin basic protein kinase (MBP kinase)
  - ribosomal S6 protein kinase (RSK kinase; i.e., a kinase that phosphorylates a kinase)
  - EGFR threonine kinase (ERT kinase).

MAP kinases act as switch kinases that transform information represented by increased intracellular tyrosine phosphorylation into serine/threonine phosphorylation.

Although MAP kinase activation is by EGF, other factors such as PDGF, nerve growth factor (NGF), insulin-like receptors, cellular stimuli such as

T-cell activation, phorbol esters (which function through activation of PKCs), thrombin, bombesin and bradykinin (which function through G-proteins), as well as the *N*-methyl-D-aspartate (NMDA) receptor may influence MAP kinases.

MAP kinases are not the direct substrates for RTKs or receptor-associated tyrosine kinases, but are in fact activated by additional classes of kinases termed MAP kinase kinases (MAPK kinases; also known as MAPK/ERK, kinases, MEKs) and MAPK kinase kinases (MAPKK kinases). One of the MAPKK kinases has been identified as the proto-oncogene serine/threonine kinase, Raf.

Targets of the MAP kinases are several transcriptional regulators, including serum response factor (SRF) and the proto-oncogene products Fos, Myc, and Jun, as well as members of the steroid/thyroid hormone receptor superfamily of proteins.

Phosphatidylinositol 3'-kinase

PI3-K is tyrosine-phosphorylated, and subsequently activated, by various RTKs and receptor-associated PTKs. It contains SH2 domains that interact with activated receptors or other receptor-associated PTKs and is itself subsequently tyrosine-phosphorylated and activated.

PI3-K associates with and is activated by PDGF, EGF, insulin, insulin-like growth factor I (IGF-I), hepatocyte growth factor (HGF) and NGF receptors. It phosphorylates various phosphatidylinositols, and this activity generates additional substrates for PLC, allowing a cascade of diacylglycerol (DAG) and inositol trisphosphate (IP_3) to be generated by a single activated RTK or other PTKs.

G-Protein-coupled receptors

There are several thousands of receptors, known as G-protein-coupled receptors (GPCRs), that couple signal transduction to G-proteins:

■ GPCRs that modulate adenylate cyclase activity. One class of adenylate cyclase-modulating receptors activates the enzyme leading to the production of cAMP as second messenger. Receptors of this class include the α-adrenergic, glucagon, and odorant molecule receptors. An increase in the production of cAMP leads to an increase in the activity of PKA in the case of α-adrenergic and glucagon receptors.

- GPCRs that activate PLC, leading to hydrolysis of polyphosphoinositides (e.g., phosphatidylinositol bisphosphate, PIP_2), and thus generating the second messengers DAG and IP_3. This class of receptors includes the angiotensin, bradykinin, and vasopressin receptors.

The activity of G-proteins is regulated by a family of proteins termed GTPase-activating proteins (GAPs). The proto-oncogene protein Ras is a G-protein involved in carcinogenesis. Regulation of Ras-GTPase activity is controlled by Ras-GAP. Several other GAP proteins besides Ras-GAP are important in signal transduction.

There are two clinically important proteins of the GAP family of proteins:

- The gene product of the neurofibromatosis type 1 (*NF1*) susceptibility locus. The *NF1* gene is a tumor suppressor gene and the protein encoded is called neurofibromin.
- The protein encoded by the breakpoint cluster region gene (*BCR*) locus. The *BCR* locus is rearranged in the Philadelphia chromosome (Ph) observed with high frequency in chronic myeloid leukemia (CML) and in some cases of acute lymphoblastic leukemia (ALL).

Intracellular hormone receptors

Hormone receptors are proteins that effectively bypass all of the signal transduction pathways by residing within the cytoplasm. Additionally, all of the hormone receptors are bifunctional. They are capable of binding hormones as well as directly activating gene transcription.

The steroid/thyroid hormone receptor superfamily (e.g., glucocorticoid, vitamin D, retinoic acid, and thyroid hormone receptors) is a class of proteins that reside in the cytoplasm and bind the lipophilic steroid/thyroid hormones. These hormones are capable of freely penetrating the hydrophobic plasma membrane. Upon binding ligands, the hormone–receptor complexes translocate to the nucleus and bind to specific DNA sequences termed hormone response elements (HREs). Binding of a complex to an HRE results in altered transcription rates of the associated gene.

Phosphatases in signal transduction

Both tyrosine and serine/threonine phosphorylation are linked with increased cellular growth, proliferation, and differentiation. Removal of the incorporated phosphates is a necessary event to turn off proliferative signals.

On the other hand, dephosphorylation may also be required in certain instances for promotion of cell growth. This is particularly true of specialized kinases that are directly involved in regulating cell cycle progression.

There are two broad classes of protein tyrosine phosphatases (PTPs):

■ Transmembrane enzymes, which contain the phosphatase activity domain in the intracellular portion of the protein. The first transmembrane PTP to be characterized was the leukocyte common antigen (LCA) protein, CD45. This protein was shown to have homology to the intracellular PTP, PTP1B. There are at least six subclasses of transmembrane PTPs.
■ Intracellularly localized enzymes. The C-terminal residues of most intracellular PTPs are very hydrophobic, suggesting that these sites are membrane-attached.

Two intracellular PTPs (PTP1C and PTP1D) have been shown to contain SH2 domains. These domains allow these PTPs to interact directly with tyrosine-phosphorylated RTKs and PTKs, thereby dephosphorylating tyrosines in these proteins.

Specific pathways

Ras pathway

■ Ras ('rat sarcoma') is a proto-oncogene product and has an effect on cellular division and growth by initiating a cascade of protein kinases that donate phosphate from ATP to particular proteins. This ultimately activates specific transcription factors to turn on transcription of target genes.
■ Ras is a member of the superfamily of G-proteins, regulated by a guanosine diphosphate (GDP)/GTP cycle. Ras is active when bound to GTP, but inactive when bound to GDP. The oncogenic form of Ras is always GTP-bound, and therefore always active. The active state of Ras is terminated by converting GTP to GDP, mediated by a GAP. Reactivation of Ras requires the removal of GDP by a guanine nucleotide exchange factor called Sos ('son of sevenless' – named after a *Drosophila* gene). Since the concentration of GTP is 10 times higher than the concentration of GDP in cells, GTP binds to unoccupied Ras.
■ Binding of growth factors to RTKs stimulates the autophosphorylation of specific tyrosines on the receptors. The phosphorylated receptor then binds to an adaptor protein called Grb2 which, in turn, recruits Sos to the plasma membrane. Sos displaces GDP from Ras, subsequently allowing the binding of GTP.

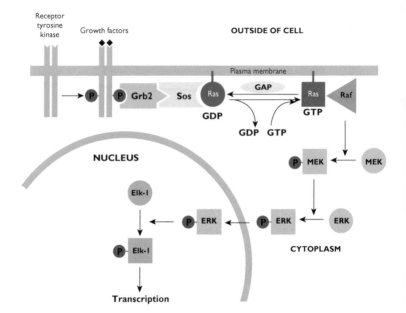

Figure 1.2 Ras pathway. GDP, guanosine diphosphate; GTP, guanosine triphosphate; GAP, GTPase-activating protein; MEK, MARK/ERK kinase; ERK, extracellular-signal regulated kinase (a nitrogen-activated protein kinase, MARK); P, phosphate group

- GTP-bound Ras recruits and activates Raf. Raf initates a cascade of protein phosphorylation by first phosphorylating MEK. Phosphorylated MEK in turn phosphorylates ERK. Phosphorylated ERK moves from the cytoplasm into the nucleus where it subsequently phosphorylates a number of transcription factors, including the specific transcription factor called Elk-1.
- Phosphorylated transcription factors turn on transcription (gene expression) of specific sets of target genes (Figure 1.2).

p53 pathway

- p53 is a tumor suppressor protein. The main role of p53 in genome stability is the removal of damaged cells when other systems fail.
- In unstressed cells, p53 is latent and is maintained at low levels by targeted degradation mediated by its negative regulator, Mdm2. Mdm2 counteracts p53 tumor suppressor activity by physically binding to p53

and suppressing its transcriptional activity. Mdm2 also functions as the p53 ubiquitin ligase and triggers its degradation. The *MDM2* gene itself is under transcriptional control by p53.

■ Activation and stabilization of p53 is by:
  – Specific protein modifications due to phosphorylation. Phophorylation prevents the binding of Mdm2 to p53 and modulates the transcriptional activity of p53.
  – Inappropriate expression of viral or cellular oncogenes, such as *RAS* or *MYC*, leads to p53 activation through a p14[ARF]-dependent pathway. p14[ARF] functions by binding to Mdm2 and neutralizing its activity. p14[ARF] inhibits the p53 ubiquitin ligase activity of Mdm2. Because the ubiquitin ligase activity of Mdm2 appears to be essential for the degradation of p53, it is possible that by directly binding and inactivating Mdm2, p14[ARF] bypasses the need for phosphorylation in p53 activation.
  – Acetylation: multiple lysine (K) residues in p53 are acetylated, stimulating its binding to DNA.

■ The p53-dependent transcription of target genes responds to a diverse range of cellular signals affecting cell proliferation and DNA integrity checkpoints:
  – In undamaged cells that are dividing normally, p53 is highly unstable, with a half-life of minutes.
  – After DNA damage induced by ionizing radiation, the half-life of p53 increases significantly, leading to accumulation of p53 and transcription of target genes such as *p21*$^{WAF1/CIP1}$ and *BAX*. The outcome is a very prolonged G_1 arrest or apoptosis.

■ p53 stimulates transcription of the CDK inhibitor gene *p21*$^{WAF1/CIP1}$, which encodes a G_1 cyclin/CDK inhibitor in response to DNA damage and leads to an S-phase delay.

■ There are several potential mediators of p53-induced apoptosis. The Bax protein is an apoptosis-inducing member of the Bcl-2 protein family. Transcription of the *BAX* gene is directly activated by p53-binding sites in the regulatory region of the gene. Bax is located in mitochondria. When overexpressed, Bax induces apoptosis.

Further reading

Adjei A, Hidalgo M. Intracellular signal transduction pathway proteins as targets for cancer therapy. J Clin Oncol 2005; 23: 5386–403.

Mani A, Gelmann E. The ubiquitin–proteasome pathway and its role in cancer. J Clin Oncol 2005; 23: 4776–89.

Shapiro G. Cyclin-dependent kinase pathways as targets for cancer treatment. J Clin Oncol 2006; 24: 1770–83.

Principles of immunology: an overview of basic immunology

A Choudhury, H Mellstedt, H Harlin
Cancer Centrum Karolinska, Stockholm, Sweden

Introduction

The immune system is a complex anatomical and functional network of cells and tissues that operate in synchrony to prevent or neutralize biological threats to the organism. Although the immune system has primarily evolved as a defense against pathogens, it may also provide surveillance and protection against the establishment of cancer.

Innate and adaptive immune system

The immune system can be primarily classified into two categories: *innate immunity* and *adaptive immunity*. Figure 2.1 schematically depicts the two categories and their interaction.

Innate immunity

- Innate immunity represents the immune components and defense mechanisms that exist inherently in the body, and does not need to be evoked or activated to become functional.
- Components of innate immunity include:
  - physical barriers such as the skin and the mucosa, which prevent the entry of pathogens, and the acidic pH of the stomach and the urinary tract, which creates a hostile environment for pathogens
  - phagocytes such as neutrophils and macrophages, which ingest pathogens and destroy them intracellularly
  - the complement system components, which can facilitate the destruction of pathogens by direct lysis or by promoting their engulfment by phagocytes.
- The innate immune system does not respond to specific antigens (immunogenic determinants), but generally reacts to a few conserved structures present on bacteria. These structures are called pathogen-associated molecular patterns (PAMPs). They include molecules such

23

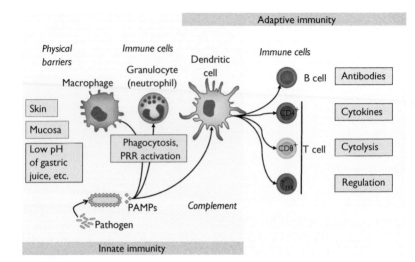

Figure 2.1 Overview of the immune system, showing the major components and effector mechanisms. The interplay between innate and adaptive immunity is illustrated. PRR, pattern recognition receptor; PAMP, pathogen-associated molecular pattern

as lipopolysaccharides, peptidoglycans, and lipoteichoic acid associated with bacteria, double-stranded (ds)RNA associated with viruses, and glucans associated with fungal cell walls. Receptors that recognize PAMPs are present on most phagocytes, and are called pattern recognition receptors (PRRs). Soluble PRRs such as mannan-binding protein (MBP), bind microbial cell wall components and in turn activate the complement system. PRRs present on phagocytes, such as CD14 on macrophages, scavenger receptors, and mannose receptors, facilitate the uptake of bacteria and their intracellular destruction in the phagocytes. Toll-like receptors are a subtype of PRRs that are found on phagocytes as well as on dendritic cells (see below) and are important signaling PRRs. Binding of microbial components to Toll-like receptors results in the triggering of intracellular signals that culminate in the secretion of soluble factors called cytokines. Many cytokines have multiple functions (i.e., are pleiotropic) and promote inflammation, migration of immune cells, and induction of adaptive immune responses. Thus, the Toll-like receptors represent a critical link between innate and adaptive immunity.

Adaptive immunity

■ Adaptive or acquired immunity represents the immune response that is specifically elicited by an antigen. Typically, the adaptive immune response has two hallmarks:

– *antigen specificity* – i.e., the immune response recognizes a particular antigen and is not generalized

– *memory* – i.e., subsequent exposure to the same antigen generates an immune response more rapidly and of greater magnitude

■ Adaptive immunity can be divided into two key sections:

– *humoral immunity*, which involves immunoglobulins or antibodies, produced by B cells

– *cell-mediated immunity*, which involves T cells.

Humoral immunity: B cells and antibodies

Almost all substances when administered as antigens in the proper context result in an antibody response. Moreover, the antibodies produced in response to an antigen or indeed even the smallest antigenic unit (epitope) can vary enormously with regard to their nature, physical properties, and binding affinity to the antigen. Despite this variety, individual monomeric antibodies are rather similar in structure and consist of two immunoglobulin (Ig) heavy chains and two Ig light chains.

There are five classes of heavy chains: α (IgA), δ (IgD), ϵ (IgE), γ (IgG), and μ (IgM). There are two types of light chains: κ and λ. Each antibody molecule is composed of only one type of light and one type of heavy chain. The heavy and light chains have constant and variable regions.

The constant region of the heavy chain determines the *isotype* of an antibody (e.g., IgM or IgA) whereas the *idiotype* of the antibody refers to the unique combination and amino acid sequence of the antibody molecule that generates its characteristic antigen-binding properties.

The diversity of the antibody repertoire results from a combination of the following processes:

■ Random somatic recombination of any of the multiple gene segments in the germline DNA that encode the constant (C), variable (V), joining (J), and diversity (D) regions of the immunoglobulin molecule

■ Imprecise joining of the gene segments that recombine during the development of a B cell

■ Somatic hypermutations acquired in the immunoglobulin sequences during differentiation of a B cell into an antibody-producing effector cell called a plasma cell

Like all other cells of the immune system, B lymphocytes are produced in the bone marrow. The recombination and rearrangement of the immunoglobulin genes occur as the B cell develops from its stem cell precursor.

All B cells initially express IgD and IgM on their surface, which act as antigen-binding receptors. Following antigenic stimulation, the first antibody produced is IgM. Subsequently the B cells undergo *isotype switching*, which results in predominant secretion of IgG. In addition to differentiating into effector plasma cells, activated B cells can also differentiate into memory B cells. Memory B cells respond rapidly to antigen and can quickly give rise to a new batch of antibody-producing cells during secondary immune responses.

Cell-mediated immunity

The cell-mediated arm of immunity is mediated by T cells. Unlike immuno-globulins, the T cell receptor (TCR) does not recognize antigen in its native state. Instead, processed antigen bound to major histocompatibility complex (MHC) molecules is presented on the surface of a cell and serves as the ligand for the TCR.

T cells are produced from pluripotent hematopoietic progenitors in the bone marrow and then undergo further differentiation in the thymus before being released as mature resting T cells. The process of 'thymic education' elimi-nates T cells with TCRs that bind self MHC molecules with too high or too low avidity. Approximately 95% of all T cells produced die in the thymus. This stringent process selects T cells that are capable of recognizing antigen in conjunction with self MHC molecules, but abrogates the possibility of autoimmune reactivity.

T cell categories

The major categories of T cells are as follows:
- *Helper T cells* are characterized by expression of the CD4 molecule on their surface. They produce cytokines that support the activation of cyto-toxic T cells and production of antibodies.
- *Cytotoxic T cells* are characterized by the expression of CD8 mole-cules. Activated cytotoxic T cells mediate cytolysis upon recognition of target cells that bear the cognate antigen and present it in the context of MHC.
- *Regulatory T cells (T_{reg} cells)* are a group of T cells that typically co-express CD4 and CD25 on their surface and express the transcription factor FoxP3. Rather than participating in the generation of an immune

response, T_{reg} cells serve as negative regulators of cell-mediated immunity and can inhibit ongoing T cell responses. T_{reg} cells are thought to play an important role in regulating autoimmunity, and have recently generated interest as a potential target for therapy in cancer immunology.

- *Memory T cells* are subpopulations of the helper and cytotoxic T cell groups and are involved in the maintenance of memory. They are generated consequent to the initial antigenic exposure and can remain dormant over a protracted period of time. They are rapidly activated following subsequent antigenic challenge, and in this way memory T cells, just like memory B cells, contribute to secondary immune responses.

Major histocompatibility complex and antigen presentation

The MHC is a critical component in the initiation of adaptive immune response, since TCRs recognize antigen only when presented in conjunction with self-MHC molecules. Figure 2.2 depicts the interaction of the TCR with the MHC.

The human MHC complex, also known as the human leukocyte antigen (HLA) complex, is composed of the A, B, and C loci, collectively called MHC class I antigens, and DP, DQ, and DR loci, which constitute MHC class II antigens.

MHC class I molecules

- These have an α chain with three domains, α_1, α_2, and α_3. The α chain is associated with another protein, called β_2-microglobulin, which is not encoded in the MHC loci.
- Exogenous antigens are presented in conjunction with class II and are recognized by helper T cells.
- The peptide-binding site of MHC class I can accommodate peptides that are eight or nine amino acids long.
- MHC class I molecules are expressed by all nucleated cells.

MHC class II molecules

- These are dimers composed of one α and one β chain, both of which are encoded by the MHC loci.
- Epitopes of intracellular proteins are presented endogenously in conjunction with class I molecules and are recognized by cytotoxic T cells.
- The peptide-binding site of MHC class II molecules can bind peptides that are 13–20 amino acids long.

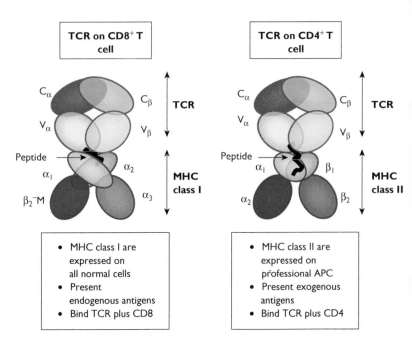

Figure 2.2 Interaction between major histocompatibility complex (MHC) class I and class II molecules, T-cell receptors (TCR), and peptide. C_α, C_β, TCR α- and β-chain constant regions; V_α, V_β, TCR α- and β-chain variable regions; α_1, α_2, α_3, β_1, β_2, MHC domains; β_2-M, β_2-microglobulin.

■ MHC class II molecules are expressed by a specialized class of cells called antigen-presenting cells (APC). Endocytosed antigens are broken down in intracellular compartments within the APC, and short peptides derived from these antigens are presented in conjunction with MHC class II. APC include macrophages, B cells, and dendritic cells (DC). Among the various APC, DC are the most potent variety and exist as a trace population in the normal human hematopoietic system. DC are the only APC that can activate naive T cells. Figure 2.3 depicts the interaction between the various molecules expressed by APC and T cells.

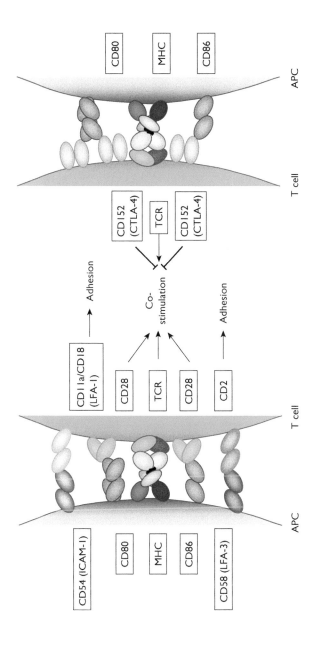

Figure 2.3 Molecules involved in co-stimulation and adhesion or in negative regulation of T-cell activation. CD28 ligation by CD80/CD86 is necessary for co-stimulation of naive T cells, whereas ligation of CD152 (CTLA-4) expressed by previously activated T cells by CD80/CD86 is important in downregulating the T-cell response. APC, antigen-presenting cell; ICAM-1, intercellular adhesion molecule I; LFA-1, -2, lymphocyte function associated antigen 1, 2; MHC, major histocompatibility complex; TCR, T-cell receptor

Tolerance and immunological anergy

In certain instances, the presentation of antigens may result in the absence of an immune response and furthermore may render the individual unreactive to subsequent challenges of the antigen. This is referred to as *tolerance*.

■ The process of thymic selection is one of the mechanisms by which the immune system is rendered tolerant to self-antigens (also called *central tolerance*).

■ Additionally, the presentation of antigen in the absence of other secondary signals, called co-stimulation, also serves to render T cells incapable of reacting to the specific antigen. This phenomenon is called *peripheral tolerance*.

■ Certain immunosuppressive cytokines, such as interleukin-10 (IL-10) and transforming growth factor β (TGF-β), as well as other factors, such as nitric oxide (NO), also promote the development of peripherally tolerized T cells.

Further reading

Abbas AK, Lichtman AH. Cellular and Molecular Immunology, 5th edn. Philadelphia: WB Saunders, 2003.

Janeway C, Travers P, Walport M, Shlomchik M. Immunobiology, 6th edn. London: Garland Science, 2004.

Principles of tumor biology

E Joosens, D Schrijvers
Ziekenhuisnetwerk Antwerpen–Middelheim,
Antwerp, Belgium

Introduction

Human carcinogenesis is a multi-step process that reflects genetic alterations, driving the progressive transformation of normal to malignant cells. The process can be arbitrarily divided into tumor initiation, tumor promotion, malignant conversion, and tumor progression. The initiation and progression to malignancy is based on the accumulation of defects or mutations in certain genes coding for certain factors. Important factors in malignant transformation are the acquired capability of:

- self-sufficiency in growth signals
- insensitivity to antigrowth signals
- evasion of apoptosis
- limitless replicative potential
- sustained angiogenesis
- tissue invasion and metastasis

It is thought that cancer cells must acquire these capabilities, although the means of acquisition may vary mechanistically and chronologically.

In addition, escape from the immune system is necessary for malignant transformation.

Gene mutations

Several types of mutation or changes in DNA have been described in cancer cells (Table 3.1). These mutations may lead to an altered protein that results in an altered function (loss or gain). In cancer cells, mutations have been seen in genes that regulate the cell cycle (proto-oncogenes and tumor suppressor genes) or repair DNA damage (repair genes).

Table 3.1 Types of mutations in cancer cells

Point mutation	Exchange of a single nucleotide for another
Insertion	One or more nucleotides or chromosomal segments are added to DNA
Deletion	One or more nucleotides or chromosomal segments are removed from DNA
Amplification	Multiple copies of a chromosomal segment
Translocation	Interchange of chromosomal segments between non-homologous chromosomes
Inversion	Reversal of the orientation of a chromosomal segment

Proto-oncogenes are genes that promote cell growth and mitosis, while tumor suppressor genes discourage cell growth or temporarily halt cell division to repair DNA. Several mutations in both types of genes have been described in cancer (Table 3.2).

Causes of mutations

Mutations in genes may be inherited or acquired during life. Mutations may be caused during life by exposure to radiation, chemicals, or viruses. If a mutation occurs in a germ cell, the germline mutation may lead to hereditary cancer.

Repair of DNA damage

The DNA mismatch repair (MMR) system is responsible for the maintenance of genomic stability. The MMR system eliminates single-base mismatches and insertion–deletion loops that may arise during DNA replication. Insertion–deletion loops result from gains or losses of short repeat units within micro-satellite sequences (microsatellite instability, MSI).

There are at least six different MMR proteins:

■ MSH2 protein forms a heterodimer with MSH6 or MSH3 for mismatch recognition:
  – MSH6 is required for the correction of single-base mispairs.
  – MSH3 and MSH6 contribute to the correction of insertion–deletion loops.

Table 3.2 Examples of mutations described in different types of cancer

Mutated gene	Type of cancer
Proto-oncogenes	
MYC	Burkitt's lymphoma
ABL	Chronic myeloid leukemia
HRAS	Bladder cancer
KRAS	Lung, colon cancer
NMYC	Neuroblastoma
ERBB2 (HER2/neu)	Breast cancer
EGFR	Squamous cell carcinoma
Tumor suppressor genes	
TP53 (p53)	Squamous cell carcinoma, colorectal cancer
PTEN	Breast, ovarian cancer
BRCA1	Breast, ovarian, colorectal, prostate cancer
BRCA2	Breast, ovarian cancer
RB1	Retinoblastoma, others
Mismatch repair genes	
MSH2, MSH6, MLH1	Heriditary non-polyposis colon cancer

■ The MLH1–PMS2 heterodimer coordinates the interplay between the mismatch recognition complex and other proteins necessary for MMR. These additional proteins may include exonuclease 1 (EXO1), helicase(s), proliferating cell nuclear antigen (PCNA), single-stranded DNA-binding protein (RPA), and DNA polymerases δ and ε.
  – PMS2 is required for the correction of single-base mismatches.
■ MLH1 may heterodimerize with two additional proteins, MLH3 and PMS1:
  – PMS2 and MLH3 both contribute to the correction of insertion–deletion loops.
  – The role of PMS1 in MMR is unclear.

If the MMR system is impaired, damage cannot be repaired and carcinogenesis may occur.

Carcinogenesis

Tumor initiation

Although irreversible genetic changes due to mutations are thought to be important initial changes in carcinogenesis, epigenetic changes may also occur as early events.

- Mutations must accumulate during DNA synthesis in proliferating cells. These DNA mutations lead to activation of a proto-oncogene or inactivation of a tumor suppressor gene.
- DNA methylation of promoter regions of genes can silence tumor suppressor genes by interfering with transcription.

Tumor promotion

Tumor promotion is the selective clonal expansion of initiated cells. Because the rate of accumulation of mutations is proportional to the rate of cell division, clonal expansion of initiated cells produces a larger population of cells that are at risk of further genetic changes and malignant conversion. This process may be influenced by tumor promoters.

Tumor promoters

- These are non-mutagenic and not carcinogenic by themselves.
- They mediate their biological effects without metabolic activation.
- They reduce the latency period for tumor formation after exposure to a tumor initiator.
- They increase the number of tumors formed.
- They induce tumor formation in conjunction with an initiator, where action is not sufficient to be carcinogenic alone.

Malignant conversion

Malignant conversion is the transformation of a preneoplastic cell into one with a malignant phenotype. This process requires further genetic changes.

Repeated exposure to a tumor promoter is important for malignant transformation, and if exposure to a tumor promoter is discontinued before malignant conversion has occurred, premalignant or benign lesions may regress.

Tumor promotion contributes to the process of carcinogenesis by expansion of the population of cells at risk for malignant conversion. Conversion of a fraction of these cells to malignancy will be accelerated in proportion to the rate of cell division and the quantity of dividing cells in the benign tumor or preneoplastic lesion.

Tumor progression

Tumor progression comprises the expression of the malignant phenotype and the tendency of malignant cells to acquire more aggressive characteristics.

Metastatic potential involves the ability of tumor cells to secrete proteases (e.g., metalloproteinases) that allow invasion beyond the immediate primary tumor location. A prominent characteristic of the malignant phenotype is the propensity for genomic instability and uncontrolled growth.

During this process, further genetic and epigenetic changes can occur, including the activation of proto-oncogenes and the functional loss of tumor suppressor genes.

The malignant phenotype

Self-sufficiency in growth signal

Normal cells require mitogenic growth signals to proliferate. These signals are transmitted by transmembrane receptors, which bind ligands such as diffusible growth factors, extracellular matrix components, and cell–cell adhesion/ interaction molecules.

In cancer cells, the dependency on growth signals is lost by alterations in the extracellular growth signals, the transcellular transducers or the intracellular circuits.

Cancer cells may:

- synthesize growth factors (autocrine stimulation), e.g., platelet-derived growth factor (PDGF) and transforming growth factor α (TGF-α)
- overexpress receptors, e.g., epidermal growth factor receptor (EGFR)
- show ligand-independent receptor activation by structural changes
- express different extracellular receptors
- contain intrinsically active intracellular pathways

Insensitivity to antigrowth signals

In normal tissues, multiple antiproliferative signals operate to maintain tissue homeostasis. These signals include soluble growth inhibitors and immobilized inhibitors embedded in the extracellular matrix and on the surfaces of surrounding cells. Antiproliferative signals are perceived by transmembrane cell surface receptors coupled to intracellular signaling circuits.

Antiproliferative signals cause:

- Transition of the cell out of the cell cycle to the resting state (G_0). Antiproliferative signals are funneled through the retinoblastoma protein (pRb) (see Chapter 1). In cancer, disruption of the pRb pathway renders the cells insensitive to antiproliferative signals.
- Cell differentiation. Cell differentiation is a complex mechanism. One of the factors of differentiation is the *MYC* oncogene. The Myc protein associates with another factor, Max. Max also associates with a group of Mad transcription factors, and this complex induces differentiation. If *MYC* overexpression is present, the balance is impaired and the Myc–Max complexes impair differentiation.

Evading apoptosis

Tumor growth is a balance between cell proliferation and programmed cell death (apoptosis). Apoptosis is a complex process, with disruption of cell membranes, extrusion of cytosol, degradation of chromosomes, and fragmentation of the nucleus.

The apoptotic machinery consists of sensors and effectors.

Sensors

- These monitor the extra- and intracellular environment for damage.
- They regulate effectors.
- They are influenced by survival (insulin-like growth factor I and II (IGF-I, -II) and interleukin-3 (IL-3)) and death factors (Fas ligand and tumor necrosis factor α (TNF-α)).

Effectors

Most pro-apoptotic signals have an influence on mitochondria, which release cytochrome *c*.

- Pro-apoptotic signal proteins are Bax, Bak, Bid, Bim, and p53.
- Anti-apoptotic signals are Bcl-2, Bcl-x_L, Bcl-w.

These signals release a number of intracellular proteases (caspases) that execute the death program through selective destruction of subcellular structures, organelles, and the genome.

Resistance to apoptosis in cancer may be by loss of a pro-apoptotic regulator (e.g., mutation of the *TP53* tumor suppressor gene) or by abrogation of the death signal (e.g., upregulation of the non-functional decoy receptor for Fas).

Limitless replicative potential

Normal cells have limited replicative potential, and, after a number of divisions, they stop growing (senescence). The mechanism of senescence is due to the limited number of telomeres, restricting the number of divisions.

Telomere maintenance is present in almost all cancer cells, by upregulation of the enzyme telomerase, which adds hexanucleotide repeats to the end of telomeric DNA.

Sustained angiogenesis

The vasculature supplies oxygen and nutrients, which are essential for cell function and survival. The growth of new blood vessels (angiogenesis) is regulated by anti-angiogenic and angiogenic factors (e.g., vascular endothelial growth factor (VEGF) and fibroblast growth factor 1 and 2 (FGF-1 and -2)).

Tumors are able to activate the angiogenic switch by changing this balance and recruit blood vessels.

Tissue invasion and metastasis

Cancer cell invasion and metastasis are due to changes in the physical coupling of cells to their microenvironment and the activation of extracellular proteases.

Interference with the microenvironment

Several classes of proteins are involved in the interaction of cells with the microenvironment, including cell–cell adhesion molecules (CAMs: e.g., immunoglobulins and cadherins) and integrins, which link cells to extracellular matrix substrates.

- E-cadherin is expressed on epithelial cells. Coupling between cells by E-cadherin bridges results in transmission of antigrowth and other signals. E-cadherin function is lost in cancer cells.
- Neural cell adhesion molecule (NCAM) is an immunoglobulin with a highly adhesive isoform that is changed to a poorly adhesive form in certain cancer types (e.g., Wilms' tumor, neuroblastoma, and small cell lung cancer) or has a reduced overall expression level (e.g. in pancreatic and colorectal cancer).

■ Growing tumor cells express different integrins that interfere with the extra-cellular matrix, enabling the cancer cells to evade control by extracellular matrix compounds.

Extracellular proteases

In cancer, protease genes are upregulated, protease inhibitor genes are down-regulated, and inactive zymogen forms of proteases are converted into active enzymes.

Conclusions

Carcinogenesis is a multistep process in which mutations lead to stepwise development of the malignant phenotype. As this complex process is under-stood in greater detail, new therapeutic approaches should become possible.

Further reading

Hanahan D, Weinberg R. The hallmarks of cancer. Cell 2000; 100: 57–70.

Fundamentals of tumor immunology

A Choudhury, H Harlin, H Mellstedt
Cancer Centrum Karolinska, Stockholm, Sweden

Introduction

The interaction between the immune system and malignancies has recently received much attention, leading to progress in immunotherapeutic approaches to cancer. Monoclonal antibodies and cytokines such as interferon-α (IFN-α) and interleukin-2 (IL-2) are now routinely used in the clinic for immunotherapy of cancers, and several tumor vaccines are in late stages of clinical development. Furthermore, in high-dose chemotherapy supported by hematopoietic stem cell transplantation, a 'graft-versus-tumor' effect mediated by allogeneic T cells in the stem cell graft is believed to play a major therapeutic role.

It is therefore imperative for those involved in cancer treatment to appreciate the critical interplay between the components of the immune system and malignant cells since the antitumor immunity of the patient is intimately linked to disease prognosis.

Immune surveillance theory

In the late 1950s, Macfarlane Burnet and Lewis Thomas proposed that the immune system contains cell populations that have the ability to recognize and destroy transformed cells before they manage to establish tumors. This theory, however, has been controversial. While this model of immune surveillance may hold for tumors of viral etiology, very little evidence could be found that non-viral-related tumors were prevented by immunosurveillance mechanisms. Animal models that lacked T and B cells did not develop spontaneous tumors at a higher frequency than immunocompetent animals.

However, more recently, information gathered from 'knockout' mice, in which a particular gene has been deleted, has led to a revival of immune surveillance theory. It has been demonstrated that recombinase activator gene (*RAG*) knockout mice that were deficient in the *STAT1* gene, and consequently had aberrant signaling of the cytokine IFN-γ, spontaneously developed gastrointestinal and lung tumors. Similarly perforin-defective mice developed spontaneous lymphomas at a high frequency.

Tumor-associated antigens

Early studies in experimental animal models with chemical carcinogen and virally induced tumors revealed that tumors were capable of spontaneously eliciting antitumor immune responses. Current techniques such as molecular cloning and gas chromatography–mass spectrometry (GC–MS) have allowed the identification of a number of molecules associated with a wide variety of cancers. These could be targeted to elicit a therapeutic immune response, and are collectively called tumor-associated antigens (TAAs).

Some of these molecules arise in tumor cells as a result of unique cellular and molecular events associated with the process of carcinogenesis. They are called tumor-specific antigens (TSAs).

Examples of TSAs are the mutated p53 and Ras proteins associated with a variety of carcinomas and the Bcr–Abl fusion proteins associated with chronic myeloid leukemia (CML).

However, in many cancers, normal cellular proteins are expressed at abnormally high levels and serve as TAAs. Examples include the HER2/*neu* (ErbB2) oncoprotein, prostate-specific antigen (PSA), and the melanoma antigen gene (MAGE) family of antigens associated with melanoma.

Viral proteins such as human papilloma virus (HPV) E6 and E7 associated with cervical carcinomas can also serve as TAAs.

Tumor immunogenicity

If tumors are immunogenic, why do they not spontaneously elicit therapeutic immune responses? There are anecdotal examples of spontaneous tumor regression after episodes of infection and fever. However, this is generally not the case and, in the absence of interventions, tumors tend to progress. There are several means by which tumors fail to generate immune responses and actually may even inhibit immune responses.

Lack of co-stimulation

The 'danger signal' model of Matzinger and Fuchs proposes that the immune system is not alerted merely by the presence of antigen, but requires a second signal, namely co-stimulation through molecules expressed on professional antigen-presenting cells (APC) such as dendritic cells (DC). These co-stimulatory molecules are expressed on DC only upon activation in the event of bacterial or viral infections, tissue damage, and inflammation. Since tumors contain largely 'self' antigens and arise without significant inflammation or tissue injury, immune responses are not evoked. Furthermore, the presentation of TAAs to T cells in the absence of co-stimulation renders them anergic to the specific antigens.

The anergy can be reversed in certain instances if the immunizing antigen is given with appropriate immunological adjuvants such as granulocyte–macrophage colony-stimulating factor (GM-CSF), bacterial cell walls or antigen-loaded DC matured ex vivo.

Immune escape mechanisms of tumors

Tumors have evolved numerous strategies to escape growth stasis and the cytolytic effects of immune effector cells.

Production of immunosuppressive cytokines

Bulky tumors are associated with systemic abnormalities in immunological function. Tumors are known to produce several immunosuppressive cytokines such as transforming growth factor β (TGF-β), IL-10, and vascular endothelial growth factor (VEGF). These cytokines have a number of effects, including:

- inhibition of T cell growth and differentiation
- induction of T cell anergy
- blocking the production of activatory cytokines
- inhibition of antigen presentation
- shift in the immune response from a T helper 1(T_{h1}) derived cytokine to a T helper 2 (T_{h2}) regulatory cell type

Production of prostaglandins, reactive oxygen species, and nitric oxide (Figure 4.1)

Tumor cells and tumor-associated macrophages produce prostaglandins, reactive oxygen species, and nitric oxide. These molecules lead to an immunosuppressive milieu in the vicinity of the tumor, and promote apoptosis and decreased function of T cells, increase vascularization, and hinder the cytotoxic activity of cytotoxic T lymphocytes (CTL).

Downregulation of MHC molecules (Figure 4.2)

Tumor cells downregulate the expression of major histocompatibility complex (MHC) molecules on their surface. This may be due to alterations in the

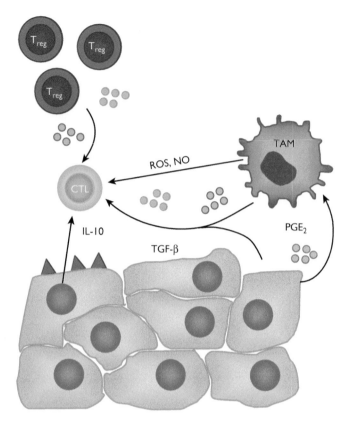

Figure 4.1 Production of prostaglandins (e.g., prostaglandin E_2 , PGE_2), reactive oxygen species (ROS), and nitric oxide (NO) by tumor cells and tumor-associated macrophages (TAM). T_{reg}, regulatory T cell; CTL, cytotoxic T lymphocyte; IL-10, interleukin -10; TGF-β, transforming growth factor β

MHC class I protein sequences that affect folding or stability, as well as to defects in the antigen-processing machinery such as downregulation of tumor-associated protein 1 (TAP1) and TAP2 which impedes presentation of endogenous antigens. The absence of functional MHC class I molecules on the surface of tumors hampers their recognition by CTL. However, tumors deficient in MHC class I may be more susceptible to lysis by natural killer (NK) cells.

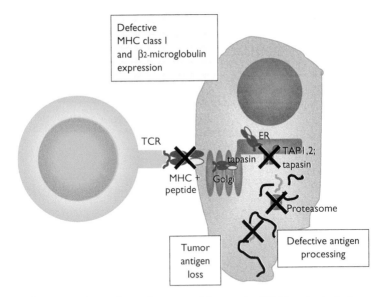

Figure 4.2 Downregulation of major histocompatibility complex (MHC) molecules by tumor cells. TCR, T-cell receptor; ER, endoplasmic reticulum; TAP 1, 2, tumor-associated protein 1, 2

Downregulation or modification of TAAs

Studies in animal models and cancer patients vaccinated with a single TAA have in several instances reported relapses due to escape variants that have modified or altogether ceased to express the targeted antigen. This immune escape is related to the inherent genetic instability of tumors, and emphasizes the need, when designing antitumor vaccines, to target cellular antigens that are essential for the survival of the tumor.

Obstruction of apoptosis (Figure 4.3)

Tumor cells frequently develop resistance to apoptosis induction by immune cells. One of the simplest mechanisms is overexpression of anti-apoptotic gene products such as Bcl-2 and v-Rel. Additionally, tumor cells can express Fas ligand which can induce apoptosis of tumor-specific lymphocytes. Expression of non-functional 'death' receptors that serve as decoys or modification of downstream components that negate the signaling of T cell ligands are also mechanisms by which tumor cells escape the induction of apoptosis.

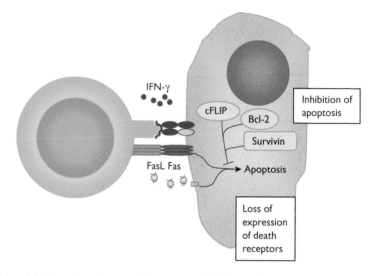

Figure 4.3 Obstruction of apoptosis by tumor cells. IFN-γ, interferon-γ; FasL, Fas ligand

Regulatory T cells and cancer

A large number of studies have established that the number of regulatory T cells (T_{reg} cells) is increased in cancer patients. In many studies T_{reg} cells are increased in the peripheral blood as well as in and around tumors. Naturally occurring T_{reg} cells are characterized as CD4$^+$ CD25$^+$ cells that also express molecules such as FoxP3 and the glucocorticoid-induced tumor necrosis factor (TNF) receptor (GITR).

The exact mechanism by which T_{reg} cells are increased in cancer is not known. It is speculated that the same antigens that generate antitumor responses may also amplify T_{reg} cells under the influence of specific cytokines or other immunomodulatory factors produced by the tumor.

Several studies have demonstrated that immune responses to cancer vaccines are increased when T_{reg} cell levels are low or have been depleted. Cyclophosphamide is one chemotherapeutic agent that is known to selectively deplete T_{reg} cells and studies in animal models as well as in patients have demonstrated that immune responses are superior when cancer vaccines are administered following pretreatment with cyclophosphamide. Other agents such as recombinant IL-2 fused to diphtheria toxin (ONTAK) for depleting T_{reg} cells are under investigation in clinical trials.

Conclusions

Comprehension of the immune defects in cancer is central not only for a better understanding of the pathophysiology of cancer but also for the development of clinically effective anticancer vaccines. Greater understanding of the individual components of this complex system and identification of methods to modulate them holds the promise of new and innovative immune therapies for cancer in the future.

Further reading

Matzinger P. Tolerance, danger, and the extended family. Annu Rev Immunol 1994; 12: 991–1045.

Self-sufficiency

M Maur, S Marsoni
Istituto Oncologico della Svizzera Italiana,
Bellinzona, Switzerland

5

Introduction

Normal cells proliferate *only* when told to do so by a variety of growth signals generated from outside the cell, which are then transmitted into the cell and conveyed to the nucleus by a complex signaling system to activate the genes for cell division. Cells, however, must also be able to stop responding to growth signals, because failure to do so could lead to uncontrolled mitosis and cancer.

Cancer cells have the means to escape these rules by using diverse strategies aimed at producing their own stimulatory growth signals and/or by deregulating the molecular machinery that processes those signals within the cell itself. These strategies are orchestrated within the cancer cell by many oncogenes that can mimic normal growth signaling.

To understand how the cancer cell can achieve growth autonomy, it is necessary to briefly recapitulate the three key players involved in growth signaling in normal cells: growth signals, growth receptors, and signaling pathways.

Growth signals

Growth signals are of different kinds, and include extracellular matrix (ECM) components, cell–cell adhesion/interaction molecules, and mostly, diffusible growth factors. There are dozens of growth factor families, such as the epidermal growth factor (EGF), transforming growth factor (TGF)-β, and vascular endothelial growth factor (VEGF). Many growth factors are versatile, stimulating cellular division in numerous different cell types, while others are specific to a particular cell-type.

Growth signals are produced, when needed, by one cell type to stimulate the proliferation of another cell type. This process is known as heterotypic signaling. The signal from the producing cell to the receiving cell can be conveyed either systemically (endocrine modulation) or by paracrine signaling, a

47

form of signaling in which the target cell is close to the signal-releasing cell and the signal is broken down chemically too quickly to be carried to other parts of the body.

Growth receptors

Growth factors bind to and activate a variety of specialized receptors on the cell surface. As a general rule, each type of growth factor binds to its own receptor and will not bind to receptors for other growth factors. For example, EGF will bind only to the EGF receptor (EGFR) but not to the VEGF receptor (VEGFR), which may also be present on the cell surface.

Growth receptors are transmembrane proteins composed of an extracellular docking region (domain) for the binding of the extracellular ligand (i.e., the corresponding growth factor), a short transmembrane domain that anchors the receptor to the cell membrane, and an intracellular effector domain with tyrosine protein kinase activity. Thus, receptors are actually enzymes, although they are not active per se (constitutively and permanently) but require to be activated by their cognate ligand.

The binding of a growth factor to the extracellular domain of its cognate receptor activates the kinase activity, usually by dimerization, starting a cascade of biochemical events:

■ autophosphorylation of specific tyrosine residues in the cytoplasmic domain at the intracellular end of the receptor
■ phosphorylation of a series of other proteins near the cytoplasmic domains that in turn become activated and thus proceed to send 'instructions' further down

Tyrosine phosphorylation is the language that receptors use to transduce the information coming from outside the cell to the cytoplasm, where it is picked up and conveyed to its ultimate destination by a complex network of signaling pathways.

Signaling pathways

Signaling pathways convey mitogenic and growth information downstream from the growth factor receptors through the cytoplasm to transcription factors in the nucleus that activate the genes for cell division. Intracellular signaling proteins include tyrosine kinases, serine/threonine kinases, phosphatases, guanosine triphosphate (GTP)-binding proteins, and many other proteins with which they interact.

The link between the receptor and the molecules of the signaling cascade is provided by a variety of molecules known as adaptor and scaffolding proteins that together with the receptor tyrosine kinase form the receptor signaling complex. Once activated, the signaling complex also undergoes autophosphorylation and then proceeds to broadcast multiple biochemical signals to a number of branching signal transduction pathways. At the end of each signaling pathway is the transcription factor protein, which is altered when the pathway is active and changes the activities of the cell.

A central role in the broadcasting program for proliferation is played by Ras. Proteins in the Ras family are molecular switches for a wide variety of signaling pathways.

An especially important pathway is the mitogen-activated protein (MAP) kinase pathway, which signals downstream to other protein kinases and gene-regulatory proteins. MAP kinases are serine/threonine kinases, and are also known as extracellular-signal regulated kinases (ERKs).

Another central player is the phosphoinositol 3'-kinase (PI3-K)/Akt-1 pathway, which can be activated directly by growth receptors or by Ras. PI3-K isoforms phosphorylate inositol lipids to form second-messenger molecules.

Self-sufficiency in cancer cells

Modulation of growth factor provision

The first strategy that cancer cells adopt for reaching self-sufficiency is to produce and secrete their own growth factors, creating a positive-feedback signaling loop termed autocrine stimulation, which is a type of autostimulation. By this strategy, tumor cells might avoid a dependence on growth factors produced by other cells within the tissue.

Examples of autocrine stimulation are secretion of platelet-derived growth factor (PDGF) by glioblastomas and sarcomas of TGF-α by sarcomas, and of granulocyte–macrophage, granulocyte, and macrophage colony-stimulating factors (GM-CSF, G-CSF, and M-CSF) in acute myeloid leukemia (AML) and overexpression of fibroblast growth factor (FGF) in prostate and breast cancers.

In addition to autocrine stimulation, cancer cells can co-opt the stromal component of their tumor mass and induce their normal neighbors to release growth-stimulating signals by paracrine signaling.

Modulation of growth factor receptor activity

The second most common mechanism of self-sufficiency is enacted at the level of growth receptors. Cancer cells can achieve autonomy by aberrant receptor activation consequent to overexpression of normal receptors or to structural alteration of the receptor resulting in ligand-independent constitutive activation of the receptor itself.

Overexpression

Overexpression of growth factor receptor RNA and/or protein, usually coupled with amplification of the gene coding for that receptor, is common in many cancers. The amplification of the receptor gene results in an increased concentration of receptor dimers at the cell membrane. This increase makes the cancer cell hyper-responsive to physiological low levels of growth factors that would not normally trigger a growth response.

A good example of this self-sufficiency strategy is HER2/*neu* overexpression/ amplification, which has been observed primarily in adenocarcinomas, especially of the breast and ovary. Overexpression of the HER2/*neu* (ErbB2) protein, amplification of the *ERBB2* gene, or both occurs in approximately 15–25% of breast cancers and is associated with aggressive behavior of the tumor. HER2/*neu* overexpression (determined by immunohistochemistry) or amplification (determined by fluorescence in situ hybridization (FISH)) is a predictive factor for response to trastuzumab (Herceptin™), a humanized monoclonal antibody against the extracellular domain of HER2/*neu,* in a metastatic and adjuvant setting. Assessment of gene amplification by FISH is the preferred method for selecting patients for trastuzumab therapy.

Overexpression of EGFR RNA and/or protein, with or without *EGFR* gene amplification, is commonly found in several solid tumors, including cancers of the upper aerodigestive tract, colon, pancreas, breast, ovary, bladder, and kidney. In non-small cell lung cancer (NSCLC), overexpression of EGFR has been reported to be present in over 50% of patients.

Gene mutations

In addition to binding of a growth factor to its cognate cell surface receptor, there are other ligand-independent mechanisms that can activate the receptor, including chromosomal translocations and mutations.

■ Chromosomal translocations can result in fusion proteins responsible for enforced dimer formation, leading to ligand-independent autophosphorylation of the receptor.

- *Chronic myelomonocytic leukemia (CMML)*. The *PDGFRB* gene on chromosome 5 encodes a cell surface tyrosine kinase receptor for members of the PDGF superfamily. These growth factors are mitogens for cells of mesenchymal origin. A translocation between chromosomes 5 and 12 that fuses this gene to that of the *TEL* ('translocation, *ETS*, leukemia') gene, results in CMML.
- *RET*. This gene, a member of the cadherin superfamily, encodes the receptor for glial-derived neurotrophic factor growth factors, and is found to be rearranged in 30% of papillary thyroid carcinomas.

■ Point mutation with gain of function in the receptor gene can also inappropriately activate the receptor in a ligand-independent fashion.
- Point mutations lead to activation of c-Kit, the receptor for stem cell factor (SCF), which is frequently found permanently activated in CML and gastrointestinal stromal tumors (GISTs).
- Activating somatic mutations of EGFR are seen in NSCLC, corresponding to the minority of patients with strong response to the tyrosine kinase inhibitors gefitinib and erlotinib.
- About 40% of gliomas express the variant III (vIII) of EGFR, in which an in-frame deletion in the extracellular domain results in a constitutively active mutant receptor that engages a broader spectrum of signal transducers than wild-type EGFR.
- Flt3 is a receptor tyrosine kinase expressed by immature hematopoietic cells and is involved in the proliferation, differentiation, and survival of early hematopoietic progenitor cells. Different types of mutations of Flt3 have been detected in about 30% of patients with AML and a small number of patients with acute lymphoblastic leukemia (ALL) or myelodysplastic syndromes (MDS). Mutation promotes ligand-independent Flt3 receptor activation.

Influencing extracellular matrix

Finally, cancer cells are also able to switch the type of ECM receptors (integrins), favoring those that transmit progrowth signals. Integrins are bifunctional, heterodimeric cell surface receptors that are linked to ECM components. Interactions between integrins and ECM components influence different functions of cell behavior, such as quiescent state, motility, apoptosis, and beginning and/or progression of the cell cycle.

Modulation of intracellular signaling pathways

The final and most complex mechanism employed by the cancer cell to acquire self-sufficiency from extracellular growth signals involves alterations in the signaling protein cascade that convey mitogenic information downstream from the growth factor receptors through the cytoplasm to the transcription factors in the nucleus that activate the genes for cell division.

Since many of these proteins are coded by proto-oncogenes that are converted into oncogenes by amplification, mutations, or translocations, it is easy to see how the signaling cascade downstream from the growth factor receptors can be continuously kept active.

RAS

Ras proteins are GTPase molecular switches for turning 'on' signaling pathways. Point mutations in the *RAS* family of proto-oncogenes (*KRAS, HRAS,* and *NRAS*) can change the Ras proteins so that they are no longer able to switch 'off', thus causing the downstream pathways to be stuck in the 'on' position.

Mutations in *KRAS* predominate in carcinomas and have been identified in cancers of many different origins, including pancreas (90%), colon (50%), lung (30%), thyroid (50%), bladder (6%), ovary (15%), breast, skin, liver, and kidney, as well as some leukemias. *NRAS* mutations are predominantly found in hematological malignancies, with up to a 25% incidence in AML and MDS, while follicular thyroid carcinomas have mutations of all three *RAS* genes.

RAF

The *RAF* oncogene encodes a serine/threonine kinase in the pathway between Ras and MAP kinase. There are three *RAF* genes in humans: *ARAF, BRAF,* and *CRAF* (also called *raf-1*). The most studied is BRAF, which is mutated in malignant melanoma (60%), papillary thyroid cancer (36–53%), colorectal cancer (5–22%), and serous ovarian cancer (30%).

Sorafenib, the first Raf kinase inhibitor, has recently been approved for the treatment of clear cell renal carcinoma. In this disease, however, the antitumor activity of sorafenib is probably due to the fact that the drug also inhibits the tyrosine kinases VEGFR-2 and PDGFR-β, key receptors of VEGF and PDGF, which play important roles in angiogenesis. Sorafenib also inhibits other receptor tyrosine kinases, such as c-Kit and Fit-3.

Signaling pathway protein tyrosine kinases are also frequent targets of somatic mutations, leading to a significant fraction of human cancers. Of the more than 100 dominant oncogenes known to date, many encode receptor and cytoplasmic protein tyrosine kinases, known to be mutated and/or over-expressed in human cancers.

CRK

The *CRK* (pronounced 'crack') oncogene encodes an adapter protein, Crk, that binds to several receptor tyrosine kinases and is a key integrator of signals involved in cell migration and invasion of highly invasive human cancer cells. Overexpression of Crk leads to formation of protein aggregates that inappropriately signal the growth and metastatic abilities characteristic of cancer cells. It is overexpressed in various human cancers, including gliomas, lung cancer, and breast cancer.

SRC

Another oncogene that encodes a constitutively active cytosolic protein tyrosine kinase is *SRC*. Phosphorylation of target proteins by aberrant Src oncoproteins contributes to abnormal proliferation of many types of cells. Src is normally found in most cells at a low level, but is overexpressed in certain cancer types, including neuroblastoma, small cell lung cancer, colon cancer, breast cancer, and rhabdomyosarcoma. Mutations in this gene could be involved in the malignant progression of colon cancer.

Conclusions

The acquisition of growth independence is a central hallmark of malignancy; however, the intrinsic and extrinsic influences that allow a normal cell to acquire this characteristic are much more complex than what has been schematically reported here.

This is partially due to the fact that much of what we know about tumor growth is derived from cell culture – an experimental model that does not take into account the stromal influence on epithelial cells. In recent years, more and more evidence has been obtained pointing toward the fact that tumors function as organs composed of many interdependent cell types, each contributing to tumor development and metastasis, and that the interactions between a tumor and its microenvironment is bidirectional and dynamic.

Stromal cells can also impart stimulatory and growth-inhibitory effects on tumor cells: for example, the malignant potential of teratocarcinoma cells can be restrained during embryonic development, resulting in cancer-free adult mice. Similarly, attenuation of β_1 integrin (laminin receptor), EGFR, or MAP kinase activation in highly aggressive human breast cancer cells results in a reversion of the aggressive phenotype.

The cell–cell and cell–matrix interactions within tumor tissue are probably as important as the cancer cell's intrinsic propensity for growth discussed above.

Further reading

Baselga J, Arteaga CL. Critical update and emerging trends in epidermal growth factor receptor targeting in cancer. J Clin Oncol 2005; 23: 2445–59.

Dhanasekaran N. Cell signaling: an overview. Oncogene 1998; 17: 1329–30.

Garnett M, Marais R. Guilty as charged: B-raf is a human oncogene. Cancer Cell 2004; 6: 313–19.

Hanahn D, Weiberg RA. The hallmarks of cancer. Cell 2000; 100: 57–70.

MIT Hypertextbook. This is a website containing the basic molecular biology that is the basis of MIT's core biology course, 'Introductory Biology': http://web.mit. edu/esgbio/www/7001main.html.

Parsons SJ, Parsons JT. Src family kinases, key regulators of signal transduction. Oncogene 2004; 23: 7906.

Robinson DR, Wu YM, Lin SF. The protein tyrosine kinase family of the human genome. Oncogene 2000; 19: 5548–57.

Vogelstein B, Winzler KW. Cancer genes and the pathways they control. Nat Med 2004; 10: 789–99.

Limitless replicative potential

M Maur, C Sessa
Istituto Oncologico della Svizzera Italiana,
Bellinzona, Switzerland

6

Introduction

An essential acquired capability of the malignant cell through which tumor tissue escapes from the mechanisms of growth control is limitless replicative potential.

After a certain period of doubling activity, normal cells in culture enter a senescence process, which ultimately leads to a crisis state with massive cell death. Tumor cells are immortalized and have the capability of unlimited replicative potential, which is acquired during tumorigenesis.

Immortalization of tumor cells is due to a balance between telomeres (special chromatin structures at the end of eukaryotic chromosomes, which shorten progressively during cellular replication, resulting in loss of telomere protection and eventual growth arrest) and telomerase (a cellular ribonucleotide enzyme responsible for adding telomere repeats at the end of chromosomes).

Telomerase is not detected in most normal tissues, with the exception of germline cells, hematopoietic progenitor cells, and cells of regenerative tissues such as the epidermis and intestinal crypts. Telomerase is reactivated or upregulated in 90% of human tumors, thus bypassing replicative senescence (Figure 6.1). Large differences in constitutive telomerase expression between most adult somatic and tumor tissues, and the critical length of telomere to be reached to trigger loss of viability in the absence of telomerase or reactivation of telomerase in tumor, indicate a window of opportunity for selective antitumor interventions.

Another process through which cancer cells acquire a limitless replicative potential or unregulated self-renewal is by cancer stem cells, which are characterized by their capacity to proliferate outside the normal growth-regulating mechanisms and to invade and destroy normal tissues.

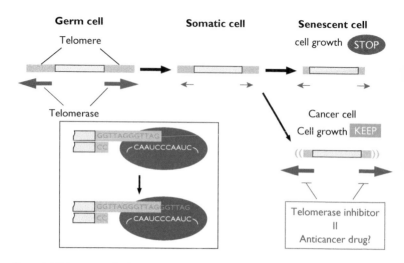

Figure 6.1 Telomere and telomerase
From Zaffaroni, 2006 (with permission)

Telomeres and telomerase

Telomere structure and function

Telomeres (Figure 6.2) are composed of repeats of TTAGGG sequences bound by specific proteins, including telomere repeat-binding factors 1 and 2 (TRF1 and TRF2; also known as TERF1 and TERF2). They are also bound by nucleosome arrays, containing histones with specific modifications of constitutive heterochromatin and with which the retinoblastoma family of proteins – retinoblastoma protein 1 (RB1, also known as pRb) and retinoblastoma-like 1 and 2 (RBL1 and RBL2) – if mutated, can interact. This provides a mechanism by which the retinoblastoma family influences telomere length and chromosome segregation.

During cell division, incomplete replication of the linear chromosome by DNA polymerase with loss of TTAGGG repeats results in loss of telomere protection, chromosomal instability, end-to-end fusion, and loss of cell viability. TRF1 regulates telomere length and function by controlling access of telomerase to the telomere; it does this through the formation of a multiprotein complex, which includes potential targets for selective antitumor treatment.

The main role of TRF2 is to protect the telomere from degradation and from DNA repair mechanisms with prevention of telomere end-to-end fusion.

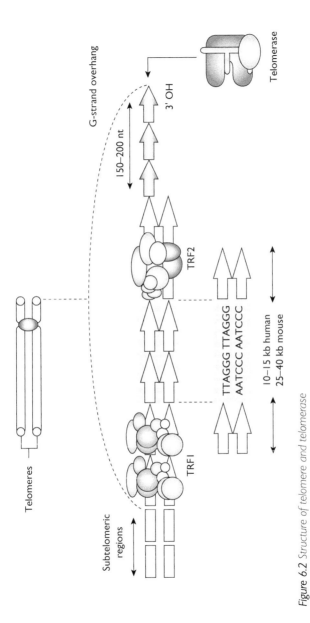

Figure 6.2 *Structure of telomere and telomerase*

From Blasco M. Telomeres and human disease: ageing, cancer and beyond. Nat Rev 2005; 6: 611–22

57

Some of the DNA repair proteins are localized at telomeres through direct interaction with TRF2. TRF2 may play a role in tumorigenesis, since it is overexpressed in many human tumors (e.g., lung, gastric, and liver cancers).

Telomerase

Telomerase is a DNA polymerase that maintains and elongates telomeres by adding de novo synthezised TTAGGG repeats to the 3′ ends of chromosomes. The two major components of human telomerase are:

- the template-containing RNA (hTR or hTERC)
- the reverse transcriptase catalytic subunit (hTERT, human transcriptase); telomerase activity is controlled by hTERT transcriptase

Targeting telomerase/telomere mechanisms (Table 6.1)

Inhibition of telomerase activity

- Inhibition of telomerase activity can be achieved by targeting the active site of hTERT with small molecules (although lack of selectivity with other polymerases might be a problem) or with non-nucleoside analogs (e.g., BIBR1532). For this class of compounds, as with other telomerase inhibitors, the long lag phase between the inhibition of telomerase and the time to telomere shortening in order to affect cellular proliferation is of concern.
- Targeting hTERT or hTR by antisense oligonucleotides might be another approach. Oligonucleotides targeting hTR might function as classical enzymatic inhibitors with activity even at a level of inhibition lower than that needed for typical mRNA targeting. After removal of the telomerase template antagonist in cell cultures, telomerase activity returns to its base-line value and telomeres to their original length, supporting the concept of a competitive inhibition of the enzyme and the need for prolonged periods of antitumor treatment. The most clinically advanced antisense-based molecule is GRN163, a 13-mer thiophosphoramidate oligonucleotide targeted at hTR.

Targeting the telomere

Telomere targeting should be very selective in order to avoid cytotoxic effects derived from non-specific interaction with other regions of the genome. Because of the ability of telomeres to fold into quadruplex intramolecular structures, tetraplex interactive compounds with a variety of pharmacophores, including antraquinones, porphyrins, acridines, fluorenones, and tetracyclic quinones, have been developed with improved selectivity.

Table 6.1 Approaches of inhibition of the telomerase/telomere system

Inhibition of telomerase activity

Inhibitors of hTR

- Antisense oligonucleotides
- Peptide nucleic acids (PNAs) [a]
- Ribozymes[b]

Inhibitors of hTERT

- Nucleotide analogs
- Antisense oligonucleotides
- Dominant-negative mutants[c]

Telomere interaction

- DNA quadruplex-interacting agents
- TRF1 interaction

[a]PNAs are complementary to the RNA component of human telomerase and induce a dose- and time-dependent inhibition of telomerase activity.
[b]Ribozymes are RNA molecules that possess specific endoribonuclease activity and catalyze the hydrolysis of specific phosphodiester bonds, resulting in cleavage of the RNA target sequences. After the cleavage reaction, the substrate is accessible by ribonucleases, a step that guarantees its permanent inactivation and offers a considerable advantage over the simple physical blockage obtained with complementary oligomers.
[c]Molecular biologists developed a new approach to assign a function to genes that have been cloned by the manipulation of these genes to create what are known as '*dominant-negative' mutations*. These encode mutant polypeptides that when overexpressed disrupt the activity of the wild-type gene. Specifically, telomerase inhibition in human tumor cell lines using dominant-negative versions of hTERT resulted in telomere shortening and cell death, suggesting that telomerase inhibition may be an effective way to halt tumor growth.

The biological activity of many G-quadruplex ligands is related to modification of the telomere capping state and rapid induction of senescence and/or apoptosis.

For the compound BRACO-19, an extensive end-to-end chromosomal fusion has been shown in tumor cell lines, with activation of the DNA damage response pathway. The latter biological effect supports the development of combinations with radiotherapy and cytotoxic agents inducing a DNA damage pathway.

Accessibility of telomerase to the telomere

The accessibility of telomerase to the telomere is controlled by TRF1. TRF1 is involved in the negative feedback regulation of telomerase, by which larger telomeres recruit more telomeric proteins that inhibit telomere elongation, such as TRF1.

Poly(ADP-ribosyl)ation of TRF1 by a telomeric poly(ADP-ribose)polymerase (PARP), tankyrase-1, causes a loss of DNA-binding activity of TRF1, with subsequent degradation and elongation of the telomere. This implies that, when used in combination with telomerase inhibitors, tankyrase-1 may confer resistance to these inhibitors and that PARP inhibitors could restore sensitivity to telomerase inhibitors.

Concerns about telomerase and telomere as anticancer agents

One potential concern with regard to the telomere/telomerase system is the lag phase between the time during which telomerase is inhibited and the time during which the telomere is shortened sufficiently in cancer cells to affect cellular proliferation. This could possibly be overcome by the development of combination regimens including other conventional or experimental cancer treatments or by the development of compounds that act as direct inhibitors of the enzyme with a more rapid biological effect.

Another concern is the potential detrimental effect on normal cells that express telomerase, such as hematopoietic progenitor cells, germline cells, and other cells of regenerating tissues. The activity of telomerase is negligible in quiescent stem cells, and the detrimental effect of telomerase inhibitors might, in general, be minor because stem cells proliferate intermittently and have much longer telomeres than cancer cells.

A third more important concern is the finding of an alternative mechanism for telomere maintenance, known as alternative lengthening of telomere (ALT) and which is derived from a process of homologous recombination-dependent replication of telomeres. Overall, ALT has so far been reported in less than 10% of tumors, but in a considerable proportion of some tumor types, including osteosarcomas and gliomas.

In general, while preclinical data on telomerase inhibitors are very promising and there is growing interest in this class of compounds, clinical data are still limited and also difficult to interpret because of the features of the compounds and the adequate but difficult methodology necessary in early clinical studies.

Cancer stem cells

Characteristics of cancer stem cells

There is evidence that tumor development may result from the clonal selection of stem cells with increasingly aggressive behavior.

Cancer stem cells have biological features comparable to those of somatic stem cells:

- *Self-renewal* – although somatic stem cells do so in a more highly regulated manner than cancer cells.
- *Differentiation* – although somatic stem cells differentiate into normal mature cells whereas cancer stem cells differentiate abnormally.
- *Organogenic capacity* – with generation of normal tissues from somatic stem cells and abnormal tissues from cancer stem cells. Tissue-specific limitations of development could be regulated by the microenvironment. Bone marrow-derived stem cells have significant plasticity and have been shown in animal models to contribute to tumor stroma and endothelium.
- *Asymmetric division* – this process results in the formation of two daughter cells (one of which is another stem cell, while the other is a committed progenitor lacking the capacity of self-renewal).

Better knowledge of the origin of cancer stem cells, and therefore of their features, could allow their identification within tumor tissues and the design of novel targeted therapies.

Origin of cancer stem cells

The cellular origin of cancer stem cells is still a matter of controversy.

- Cancer stem cells might arise from cell–cell fusion between one or more mutated cells (Figure 6.3). Numerous species-specific and cell-type-specific fusogenic factors have been identified. Horizontal gene transfer with DNA delivery from donor to recipient genome, incorporation, and expression have been shown to be responsible for antibiotic resistance in bacteria and in general for some acquired mutations. Horizontal gene transfer involves transferring fragmented DNA from donor apoptotic cells, previously mutated, to recipient cells by phagocytosis, followed by incorporation into the genome and expression in a beneficial manner for the recipient (Figure 6.4).

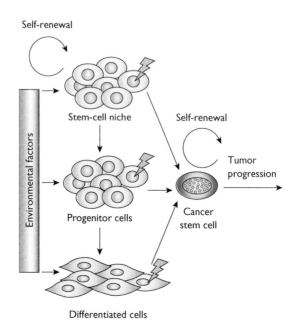

Figure 6.3 Origin of cancer stem cell

From Bjerkvig R, Tysnes BB, Aboody KS, Najbauer J, Terzis AJA. The origin of the cancer stem cell: current controversies and new insights. Nat Rev Cancer 2005; 5: 899–904

■ Mutations are essential in the pathogenesis of cancer, and they could involve stem cells or restricted progenitors or differentiated cells, which acquire properties of cancer stem cells.

■ Committed progenitor cells that do not have the capacity of self-renewal might also be transformed through the activation of oncogenic pathways that re-establish properties of self-renewal.

■ A hypothetical model depicting the organization of stem cells in normal organs and tumors has also been described. Normal stem cells are located in a highly organized stem cell niche and are regulated by paracrine signals derived from the niche cells or the extracellular matrix (ECM) components as well as by circulating hormones. On the other hand, cancer stem cells and their progeny are randomly distributed in a cancer stem cell niche where differentiated and/or stromal cell coexist. The whole ECM of cancer might function as specialized 'niche' ECM.

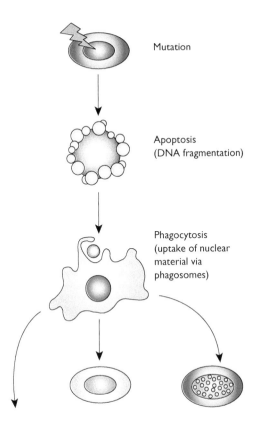

Mutation

Apoptosis
(DNA fragmentation)

Phagocytosis
(uptake of nuclear
material via
phagosomes)

Figure 6.4 Horizontal gene-transfer phenomena

From Bjerkvig, R, Tysnes, BB, Aboody, KS, Najbauer J, Terzis AJA. The origin of the cancer stem cell: current controversies and new insights. Nat Rev Cancer 2005; 5: 899–904

Evidence for cancer stem cells

Evidence for cancer stem cells was first documented in hematological malignancies, where only a small subset of cancer cells was capable of forming new tumors. Using in vivo models in which acute myeloid leukemia (AML) cells were transplanted into immunodeficient mice, a leukemia-initiating cell with a CD34+CD38− phenotype and strikingly immature features was identified.

Cancer stem cells in solid tumors have been much more difficult to identify than in hematological malignancies because fewer well-characterized phenotypic markers are available: for example, glioblastomas, medulloblastomas, and astrocytomas contain cells that may be multipotent neural stem cell-like cells (NSCs), showing immunoreactivity for nestin and CD133.

Recently, a putative breast cancer stem cell-like population, defined by the presence or absence of two cell surface markers (CD44, an adhesion molecule that binds hyaluronate, and CD24, an adhesion molecule that binds P-selectin) has been identified. This CD44$^+$CD24$^{-/low}$lineage$^-$ cell population lacks differentiated breast epithelial cell-lineage markers and has a 10–50-fold increased ability to form tumors in xenografts compared with the bulk of breast tumor cells.

Pathways in cancer stem cells

Recent data suggest that many signaling pathways involved in normal stem cells renewal are dysregulated in human cancers because of mutations. The main pathways involved are Wnt, PTEN, transforming growth factor β (TGF-β), Hedgehog, Notch, Hox and BMI-1.

■ Wnt are secreted proteins that bind to receptors called Frizzleds, which cause β-catenin to accumulate and translocate into the nucleus, where it binds to the LEF/TC transcription factors and activates the transcription of genes promoting proliferation. Mutations of Wnt/β-catenin have been reported in colon, prostate, and ovarian cancers. Ectopic activation of Wnt might induce cancer proliferation by overactivating the self-renewal program. An example may be the hyper-self-renewal of normal stem cells caused by mutation of intestinal crypt stem cells, with generation of benign polyps; additional mutations confer malignancy and allow cancer progression. Hematopoietic stem cell self-renewal is also promoted by Wnt signaling. However, it is still not clear if Wnt mutations are required for the genesis or progression of leukemia.
■ Other signaling pathways involved in dysregulated cancer stem cell renewal are reported in Table 6.2.

Therapeutic implications

Targeting cancer stem cells is crucial for controlling tumor growth, particularly in leukemia and other hematological malignancies, in which the requirement for self-renewal is absolute and more critical than in solid tumors. Chemotherapy targets the majority of the non-clonogenic tumor cells but spares leukemia stem cells, leading to relapse.

Identifying self-renewal genes through microarray studies could allow the design of agents or combinations with chemotherapy that could kill cancer

Table 6.2 Signaling pathways, stem cells and cancer

Pathway	Stem cell	Cancer
Wnt	Hematopoietic	ALL
	Intestinal epithelial	Colorectal
	Keratinocyte	Pilomatricoma
	Cerebellar granule cell progenitors	Medulloblastoma
	Central nervous system	Gliomas?
Sonic hedgehog (SHH)	Hair-follicle progenitors	Basal cell carcinoma
	Cerebellar granule cell progenitors	Medulloblastoma
	Central nervous system	Gliomas
BMI1	Hematopoietic	B-cell lymphomas
		AML
Notch	Hematopoietic	ALL
	Mammary epithelial	Breast cancer
PTEN	Neural	Gliomas

ALL, acute lymphoblastic leukemia; AML, acute myeloid leukemia;
PTEN, phosphatase and tensin homolog deleted from chromosome 10.
Adapted from Pardal R, Clarke MF, Morrison SJ. Applying the principles
of stem-cell biology to cancer. Nat Rev Cancer 2003; 3: 895–902.

stem cells. In addition, unknown features differentiating between stem cells
of different cancers could improve diagnosis, classification, and treatment.

Overcoming drug resistance

One particularly intriguing property of stem cells is that they express high levels of the specific ATP-binding cassette (ABC) drug transporters, which make
cancer stem cells more resistant to chemotherapeutic agents. The two ABC
transporters most widely studied are ABCB1, which encodes P-glycoprotein,
and ABCG2. The drug-transporting property of stem cells conferred by ABC
transporters is the basis for the 'side-population' (SP) phenotype, which is
identified by exclusion of the fluorescent dye Hoechst 3342. Stem cells are
predominantly found in the SP fraction, but SPs have also been identified in
breast cancer, lung cancer, and glioblastoma cell lines. Obviously, not only

stem cells but also differentiated tumor cells are inherently drug-resistant, so that therapies have little or no effect – as shown in renal cell cancer, in which ABCB1 is expressed in all cells and contributes to chemotherapy resistance. Taking this into account, it might be possible to overcome drug resistance by combined treatment with cytotoxic agents and ABC-transporter inhibitors.

Stem cell inhibitors

Other therapeutic opportunities might be stem cell inhibitors (e.g., cyclopamine, a compound that inhibits the Hedgehog–Patched receptor signaling protein Smoothened).

Targeting cancer stem cell self-renewal

Drugs that induce differentiation of cancer stem cells or that inhibit, even transiently, the maintenance of the stem cell status could result in conversion of malignant to benign tumors due to exhaustion of the pool of cancer stem cells.

Drugs selective for cancer stem cells

Cancer stem cells are likely to be more dependent on some pathways than normal stem cells, even if these pathways are active in both. Some agents that are selectively directed against cancer stem cells without undue toxicity to normal stem cells are being evaluated.

Further reading

Bjerkvig R, Tysnes BB, Aboody KS, Najbauer J, Terzis AJA. The origin of the cancer stem cell: current controversies and new insights. Nat Rev Cancer 2005; 5: 899–904.

Blasco M. Telomeres and human disease: ageing, cancer and beyond. Nat Rev Cancer 2005; 6: 611–22.

Folini M, Zaffaroni N. Targeting telomerase by antisense-based approaches: perspectives for new anti-cancer therapies. Curr Pharm Des 2005; 11: 1105–17.

Kelland LR. Overcoming the immortality of tumor cells by telomere and telomerase based cancer therapeutics-current status and future prospects. Eur J Cancer 2005; 41: 971–9.

Pardal R, Clarke MF, Morrison SJ. Applying the principles of stem-cell biology to cancer. Nat Rev Cancer 2003; 3: 895–902.

Seimiya H. The telomeric PARP, tankyrases, as targets for cancer therapy. Br J Cancer 2006; 94: 341–5.

Shay JW, Wright WE. Telomerase: a target for cancer therapeutics. Cancer Cell 2002; 2: 257–65.

Regulation of apoptosis

7

L Pleyer, I Tinhofer, R Greil
Paracelsus Medical University, Salzburg, Austria
G Damia, S Marsoni
SENDO Foundation, Milan, Italy

Introduction

Homeostasis of tissues is regulated by a balance between cell death and cell proliferation. Disturbances in this rheostat of cellular turnover may contribute significantly to carcinogenesis. Pathological longevity of cells is a consequence of blocks in programmed cell death (apoptosis). Apoptosis is an evolutionarily conserved form of controlled cellular self-destruction, in contrast to necrosis, which is a form of cell death consequent to acute cellular injury.

Apoptosis has many important physiological functions:

■ It is essential for successful embryonic development and for maintenance of normal cellular homeostasis. During development, many cells are produced in excess and are eliminated through apoptosis:
  – In a developing embryo, the cells between the fingers undergo apoptosis so that the fingers can separate.
  – In the fetal brain, half of the original neurons die in later stages when the adult brain is formed.
■ Tissue homeostasis relies on apoptosis to eliminate cells that have completed their life cycle, as in the skin, intestinal mucosa, and blood cells.
■ Apoptosis also plays a pivotal role in the regulation of the immune system: ineffective cells (the majority of freshly made T lymphocytes fail to connect with foreign antigens) and those showing high affinity for self-antigens are committed to death through apoptosis, allowing tight control over the pool of highly efficient but not self-reactive immune cells.
■ When cells are infected by a virus or damaged beyond repair, apoptosis can either be triggered by the cell itself or be 'commanded' by signals from the surrounding tissues and/or from immunocompetent cells.

■ Apoptosis is also triggered by diverse stress conditions, such as starvation or damage to the cell's DNA resulting from exposure to ultraviolet or ionizing radiation, or by toxicity induced by cytotoxic drugs.

Given all of these important physiological functions, it is not surprising that apoptosis is implicated in various pathological conditions such as cancer, autoimmunity, and persistent infections. In fact, excessive apoptotic signaling causes cell loss and contributes to neurodegenerative diseases (e.g., Alzheimer's disease, Parkinson's disease, and Huntington's disease), autoimmunity, acquired immunodeficiency syndrome (AIDS), and ischemia. Defective apoptosis results in uncontrolled cell proliferation, and plays a pivotal role in tumor pathogenesis and drug resistance. In recent years, it has become apparent that tumorigenesis is the ultimate outcome of both excessive proliferation driven by oncogenes and defects in apoptosis due to impairment in apoptotic pathways.

Molecular mechanisms of apoptosis

Cells undergoing apoptosis shrink and fragment, forming apoptotic bodies without bursting the cell membrane. These bodies are then engulfed by macrophages and removed from the tissue without spillage of their internal contents into the extracellular space, thus avoiding triggering an inflammatory response as happens with necrosis. These morphological modifications are the consequence of characteristic molecular and biochemical events, most notably the activation of proteolytic enzymes (caspases).

The biochemical and molecular mechanisms of the apoptotic process have recently been unravelled. Apoptosis can be induced through two signaling pathways: the extrinsic (or death receptor) pathway and the intrinsic (or mitochondrial) pathway (Figure 7.1). The former is triggered by the binding of an extracellular ligand to a receptor located on the plasma membrane, whereas the latter, which is the major form of apoptosis in human cells, is usually activated in response to intracellular stress signals, including DNA damage, reactive oxygen species, viral infection, and oncogene activation.

Caspases

Both pathways converge in the activation of a family of cysteine proteases – the caspases – that, cleaving different substrates, leads to the previously described morphological changes.

There are two types of caspases: *initiator caspases* (caspases-8–10) cleave inactive proforms of effector *caspases* (caspases-3, -6, and -7), which in this

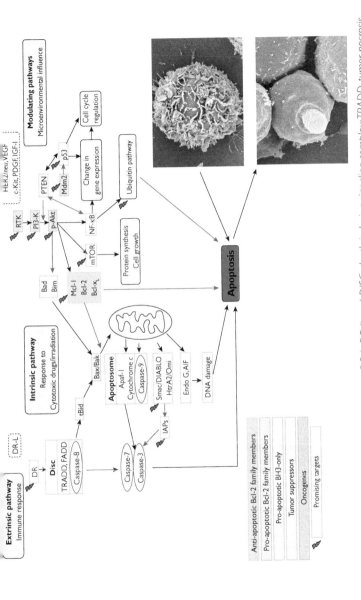

Figure 7.1 Apoptotic pathways. DR, death receptor; DR-L, DR ligand; DISC, death-inducing signaling complex; TRADD, tumor necrosis factor receptor-associated death domain; FADD, Fas-associated death domain; Apaf-1, apoptotic protease activating factor; RTK, receptor tyrosine kinase; PI3-K, phosphatidylinositol 3'-kinase; NF-κB, nuclear factor κB; VEGF, vascular endothelial growth factor; PDGF, platelet-derived growth factor; IGF-1, insulin-like growth factor I

way become activated and cleave other protein substrates within the cell, 'executing' the apoptotic process. The signaling cascade mediated by caspases, once activated, is irreversible and therefore requires a fine-tuned regulation to prevent its inappropriate and untimely triggering. Direct inhibitors of the caspases are the inhibitors of apoptosis proteins (IAPs).

Death receptors and the extrinsic pathway

The extrinsic pathway is initiated by the binding of a ligand to transmembrane receptors, called death receptors. Both receptors and ligands belong to the tumor necrosis factor (TNF) superfamily. The extrinsic pathway is used by T cells and natural killer (NK) cells to eliminate (pre)neoplastic and virally infected malignantly transformed cells

Death receptors are characterized by an extracellular domain and an intracellular death domain, which is essential for transduction of the apoptotic signal.

There are several death ligands: the major extrinsic mediator of apoptosis is TNF, a cytokine produced mainly by activated macrophages; another important mediator is the Fas ligand (FasL), a cell surface molecule expressed predominantly on NK cells and activated T cells.

The binding of the ligand to the receptor results in the formation of a death-inducing signaling complex (DISC), which contains the death domain of the receptor, an adaptor molecule (FADD: Fas-associated death domain), and the initiator caspases-8 and/or -10, and in which the initiator caspases are activated. After DISC formation, the execution of apoptosis follows two different pathways, depending on the cell type. In type I cells, the death signal is directly propagated by the active caspase-8 to the executioner members of the caspase family. In type II cells, DISC formation results in activation of caspase-8 and recruitment of the intrinsic pathway, with amplification of the pathway.

Mitochondria and the intrinsic pathway

The intrinsic pathway is used by cells to respond to cellular damage induced by cytotoxic agents and/or irradiation. This form of apoptosis is also called the mitochondrial pathway, because it is initiated and orchestrated by mitochondria. The mitochondria act as integrating sensors of different death stimuli mediated by Bcl-2–BH3 proteins, leading to mitochondrial outer membrane permeabilization (MOMP). When MOMP occurs, there is a sudden release into the cytosol of proteins normally found in the space between the inner and outer mitochondrial membranes. One of the proteins released is cytochrome c, an important component of the mitochondrial respiratory chain, which, once translocated in the cytosol, stimulates the assembly of a multiprotein complex, called the apoptosome. The apoptosome serves as a platform to recruit and activate the initiator caspase-9, which starts the activation of effector caspases, leading to cell death. MOMP can promote cell death in addition through the release of molecules involved in caspase-independent cell death, and the loss of mitochondrial functions essential for cell survival. MOMP is believed to be a 'point of no return' in the mitochondrial apoptotic pathway, and is regulated by Bcl-2 family proteins.

Apoptotic regulatory pathways

Many, if not all, types of cancer are characterized by defects in apoptotic regulatory pathways, such as p53, nuclear factor kB (NF-kB), the ubiquitin–proteasome system, and phosphatidylinositol 3′-kinase (PI3-K)/Akt.

p53

Acquired mutations in the *TP53* gene encoding the p53 protein or the p53 pathway are found in all major types of human cancer at an incidence of at least 50%. As a transcription factor, p53 controls DNA repair, passage through the cell cycle and induction of – as well as sensitivity to – apoptosis via multiple distinct pathways in response to genotoxic events, in a cell type- and signal-specific manner. This is achieved through:

- activation of genes in both the extrinsic pathway (via upregulation of death receptors) and the intrinsic pathway (through transcriptional induction of pro-apoptotic and repression of anti-apoptotic Bcl-2 family members)
- activation of REDOX genes (thereby inducing/facilitating mitochondrial pore opening)
- negative regulation of PI3-K signaling through activation of the PTEN tumor suppressor (which also protects p53 from MDM2)

p53 also mediates apoptosis in a transcription-independent manner via mitochondrial accumulation, with direct activation of Bax and Bak.

The Bcl-2 family

Bcl-2 is a superfamily of both pro-apoptotic and anti-apoptotic proteins. All members share at least one of four characteristic domains of homology called Bcl-2 homology domains (BH1, 2, 3, 4). The balance between the pro- and anti-apoptotic members of this superfamily governs the mitochondrial permeability, promoting or preventing the formation of pores. The apoptotic process is initiated by the members of the BH3-only pro-apoptotic family in response to different stress signals (which member of the BH3-only subfamily has the honor of being the initiator depends on the kind of stress). Once activated, the BH3-only proteins interact with the multidomain pro-apoptotic proteins Bax and Bak, inducing the activation of MOMP, release of cytochrome c, and caspase activation. The death signal can be interrupted by the anti-apoptotic Bcl-2 subfamily members (Bcl-2/Bcl-x_L) that can bind and sequester the BH3-only family members and also Bax and Bak, and in this way the entire system is kept under control. Another pro-apoptotic protein also released from the mitochondria is Smac/DIABLO. Smac/DIABLO facilitates apoptosis by neutralizing the IAPs, which are physiological intracellular inhibitors of caspases.

NF-κB

The transcriptional regulator NF-κB not only controls the expression of numerous genes involved in immune or inflammatory responses and cellular proliferation, but also promotes tumorigenesis by protecting cancer cells from apoptosis via induction of anti-apoptotic proteins such as the IAPs and Bcl-x_L.

NF-κB is regulated at the protein level by:

- phosphorylation (which is often constitutively aberrant as a hallmark of cancer)
- proteasomal degradation
- increased activity of histone deacetylases (HDACs) on the genetic level, which are required co-activators of NF-κB-dependent transcription

Deregulation of NF-κB is commonly augmented further by induction/activation following cytotoxic treatment, which is counterproductive since it suppresses the apoptotic potential of chemotherapeutic agents and contributes to chemoresistance. Therefore, targeting of NF-κB by inhibitors of the proteasome and/or HDACs can prevent tumor resistance and increase the efficacy of many anticancer agents.

Ubiquitin–proteasome system

The proteasome is part of the ubiquitin–proteasome pathway, which plays an essential role in the degradation of cell cycle regulators, transcription factors (e.g. p53, Mdm2, and NF-κB), and Bcl-2 family members, all of which are relevant to cancer initiation and progression, as well as drug resistance.

Inhibition of the proteasome leads to cell cycle arrest in normal cells (which resume proliferation once proteasome activity is restored) and apoptosis in transformed cells. The latter often display dysfunctional checkpoint mechanisms, rendering them more susceptible to proteasome-inhibitor-induced apoptosis.

Proteasome inhibition results in apoptosis via:

- p53 activation and stabilization
- downregulation of anti-apoptotic proteins (FLIP, IAPs, and Bcl-2 family members)
- increasing pro-apoptotic activity of BH3-only proteins
- upregulation of cell surface death receptor and/or death receptor ligand expression
- inactivation of NF-κB

The latter leads to inhibition of angiogenesis and metastasis formation via downregulation of NF-κB-induced expression of vascular epithelial growth factor (VEGF), cell adhesion molecules, growth factors, and cytokines.

The PI3-K/Akt pathway

PI3-K/Akt-signaling plays a central role in cell survival, proliferation, motility, and neovascularization. Aberrant hyperactivation is commonly genetically selected during tumorigenesis and provides the basis for a reasonable therapeutic index of inhibitors of this pathway.

Akt functions as a cardinal nodal point for converging upstream signaling pathways involving receptor tyrosine kinases, such as the well-known HER2/*neu* (c-ErbB2) receptor, VEGFR, c-Kit, the platelet-derived growth factor receptor (PDGFR) and the insulin-like growth factor I receptor (IGF-IR). These receptors recruit PI3-K and subsequently Akt to the membrane. Activated Akt then promotes survival by inhibiting transcription or activity of pro-apoptotic proteins (e.g., p53, Bad, and procaspase-9), as well as activating prosurvival proteins (such as NF-kB). Akt also regulates cell cycle progression and stimulates protein synthesis and cell growth via activation of the mTOR ('mammalian target of rapamycin') pathway (Figure 7.1). Akt-independent contributions of PI3-K to tumorigenesis include stimulation of metastasis by increasing cell motility and angiogenesis.

Malfunction in apoptosis and cancer

Evasion of apoptosis is one of the essential alterations in cell physiology leading to malignant transformation, and it is a hallmark of most, if not all, tumors. Dysfunction in the apoptotic process has also been associated with resistance to chemo/radiotherapy, as most chemotherapeutic agents work by inducing apoptosis.

In many cancers, pro-apoptotic genes carry inactivating mutations, while anti-apoptotic genes are often upregulated, leading to unchecked tumor growth and the inability to adequately respond to cellular stress and DNA damage. *BCL2* (encoding Bcl-2) was the first anti-apoptotic gene found to be overexpressed in a variety of cancer types (especially lymphomas and melanomas); on the contrary, the genes encoding the pro-apoptotic Bax and Bak have been found to be downregulated in colon and gastric cancers.

Malfunction of apoptosis in cancer cells also largely depends on gene mutations that indirectly regulate the apoptotic machinery. The most important and widely studied gene bearing on apoptosis is the tumor suppressor gene *TP53*, which is found to be mutated in more than half of human tumors. Its product p53 acts as a transcriptional factor: under unstressed conditions, its cellular levels are very low, as it is degraded by binding with another protein called Mdm2. Upon oncogene activation, hypoxia, and especially DNA damage, p53 accumulates and activates a number of different target genes that commit the cell either to cell cycle arrest and DNA damage repair or, if the damage is not reparable, to apoptosis. Because of this key role, p53 is often referred to as the 'cellular gatekeeper for life and death'. The commitment to apoptosis is carried out by p53 by stimulating the expression of several pro-apoptotic proteins (Bax, Puma, NoxA, Apaf-1, Fas, and DR5) or by repressing the expression of anti-apoptotic proteins (Bcl-2, Bcl-X_L, and survivin). It should be noted that most chemotherapeutic agents used in the treatment of cancer can induce p53 (because they induce DNA damage).

On the other hand, apoptosis can be suppressed by an overabundance of growth signaling cascades from (mutated/overexpressed) growth factor receptors along the major survival pathways down to the PI3-K/Akt signal transduction pathway. This pathway mediates a number of anti-apoptotic mechanisms, including inhibition of p53 (through phosphorylation and activation of its inhibitor Mdm2) or by direct inactivation of Bad and caspase-9, as well as other mechanisms.

Current and promising therapeutic options in apoptosis modulation

Targeting death-receptor-mediated apoptosis

Restriction to the tumor area is a *conditio sine qua non* in order to reduce systemic toxicity of death receptor activation by recombinant ligands or activating antibodies to acceptable levels. Tumor-specific targeting has been attempted via recombinant production of soluble death ligands either as trimeric fusion proteins or coupled to prodrugs, or gene therapy with cell-specific promoters. Convincing results with tumor eradication and enhanced survival have been achieved with trimeric death receptor ligand variants combined with cytotoxic drugs in murine models. Tumor selectivity has been explained by higher expression of decoy receptors in normal cells than in tumor cells, but is not completely understood.

Targeting the intrinsic death pathway

Targeting Bcl-2 family members

Strategies for targeting anti-apoptotic Bcl-2 family members include the use of:

- antisense oligonucleotides that recognize their mRNA (e.g., Genasense)
- sensitizing and activating BH3 peptidomimetics
- kinase inhibitors (e.g., flavopiridol) that inhibit their activity
- modulation of their transcription via modulation of PTEN, NF-κB, Akt, or FOXO

Targeting the mitochondria

A recurrent problem with conventional cytotoxic agents is that their effects on induction of apoptosis can be compromised by alterations in the extrinsic, intrinsic, or apoptosis-modulating pathways (Figure 7.1). Therefore, one should combine therapies that simultaneously stimulate different pathways in order to preclude resistance emerging from targeting of merely one pathway. Alternatively, targeting of more downstream events of the common apoptotic pathway in which most types of pro-apoptotic signals converge (e.g., IAPs) should prove highly useful in killing resistant tumor cells.

In principle, there are two pharmacological approaches targeting the intrinsic pathway:

- inhibition of Bcl-2 family proteins, which exquisitely control mitochondrial pore formation
- direct targeting of specific mitochondrial pore components (e.g., ANT, VDAC, PBR, and Cyp-D), which has already demonstrated selective cytotoxicity towards transformed cells as well as chemosensitizing effects with improved response rates, time to progression, and survival in phase II and III clinical trials

The challenge is now to selectively target these agents to mitochondria of malignant cells, in order to prevent central nervous system and other organ toxicity. This can be achieved by:

- exploiting differences in composition and/or regulation of mitochondrial pores between tumor cells and normal cells
- fusion of mitochondriotoxic motifs to targeting peptides that selectively bind to and are taken up by tumor cells (e.g., KLAKLAK or interleukin-2 (IL-2)/Bax fusion proteins)

Targeting apoptosis-modulating pathways

Targeting p53

As both activation and reversible suppression of p53 can be useful for cancer treatment, and p53 activity is tissue-specific, the role of p53 in tumor treatment is not as simple as was initially assumed. Apparently, the risk/benefit ratio of p53 modulation varies according to the underlying malignancy. Preferential reactivation of mutant p53 in tumor cells contributes to more efficient tumor cell killing (through reactivation of chemo/radiotherapy-mediated p53-dependent apoptosis), and leads to reversion to a much less aggressive tumorigenic phenotype.

Although activation of p53-dependent apoptosis is viewed as a promising anticancer strategy, it can also account for considerable toxicity of radio- and chemotherapy. Accordingly, it has been proposed that inhibitors of p53-mediated apoptosis be used to transiently inhibit apoptosis (and thus treatment-related side-effects) in normal tissue during high-intensity regimens. Furthermore, initial evidence suggests that p53 may play a protective role in tumor endothelium, thus defining a new potential application of p53 inhibitors as anti-angiogenic supplements of chemo/radiotherapy. Importantly, temporary reversible inhibition of p53 seems to be relatively safe compared with total p53 deficiency, which is associated with a high incidence of treatment-resistant tumors. Additionally, p53 inactivation even seems to chemosensitize tumors that lack p53-dependent apoptosis (which is mediated via activation of Bax, Puma, and NoxA, as well as direct translocation of p53 to the mitochondria) but retain p53-dependent growth arrest (mediated through induction of p21 or 14-3-3-σ). This, and the fact that p53 activation causes growth arrest in non-transformed cells and apoptosis in tumor cells, renders the development of small-molecule modulators specific for either the growth-inhibitory or pro-apoptotic functions of p53 a particularly promising approach.

Targeting MDM2

Targeting of MDM2 can be based on inhibitory small molecules, which either target the binding of Mdm2 to p53 or the activity of MDM2 as E3-ligase. Furthermore, Mdm2-specific antibodies or the knockdown of *MDM2* gene expression via small interfering RNA (siRNA) or antisense oligonucleotides (ASOs) are in development.

Targeting NF-κB via HDAC and proteasome inhibition

HDAC inhibitors induce a small set of genes resulting in growth arrest, terminal differentiation, can trigger both intrinsic apoptosis and caspase-independent autophagic cell death, exhibit potent anti-angiogenic and antimetastatic properties as well as high tumor selectivity, and have been found to be additive and synergistic with a number of anticancer agents, including TRAIL (tumor necrosis factor-related apoptosis-inducing ligand) and proteasome inhibitors. Unlike direct proteasome inhibitors (e.g., bortezomib), which target the active sites of the proteasome, HDAC inhibitors suppress proteasome activity indirectly, and also suppress NF-κB by several mechanisms.

In addition, HDAC inhibitors also have the potential to reverse silenced genes, thus allowing reactivation of tumor suppressor genes that had been silenced by hypoacetylation during tumorigenesis.

Although proteasome-inhibition-mediated blockage of NF-κB activation has already demonstrated safety and efficacy in phase III/IV clinical trials, selective inhibition of HDAC isoenzymes, NF-κB-activating kinases, or selective targeting NF-κB subunits might be more specific and generate fewer side-effects. However, many proteins and pathways involved in apoptosis have redundant functions and are involved in both the extrinsic and intrinsic pathways. Thus, selective blockers may not be enough to induce apoptosis, which, combined with the ability of both proteasome and HDAC inhibitors to influence proteasome function, provides the rational for combination therapies.

Targeting PI3-K/Akt

Blocking of the PI3-K/Akt pathway simultaneously inhibits proliferation of tumor and vascular cells and sensitizes the former to chemotherapy-induced apoptosis. Inhibition can be achieved indirectly by intervening upstream of PI3-K with kinase inhibitors (e.g., trastuzumab, imatinib, erlotinib, and gefitinib), or by direct targeting of PI3-K, isoforms, Akt, or downstream components such as Bad, FOXO proteins, or mTOR.

However, therapeutic success can be hampered by activating mutations or gene amplifications affecting downstream signaling components, or by loss of negative regulators such as PTEN. The *PTEN* gene is among those most commonly mutated in human malignancy and confers resistance to receptor tyrosine kinases (RTKs) by:

- setting a high threshold of Akt activation and consequently modulating mTOR activity
- activating transcriptional activity of antiapoptotic NF-κB
- inhibiting pro-apoptotic FOXO-mediated transcription

Downregulation of Akt by a pharmacological approach (PI3-K inhibitors and PTEN mimetics) or a genetic approach (dominant-negative Akt) enhances p53 transcriptional activity and resensitizes tumor cells to death receptor-mediated and/or RTK inhibitor-mediated apoptosis, as well as to ionizing radiation and p53-inducing drugs. The mTOR inhibitors rapamycin (sirolimus, CCI-779) and everolimus (RAD001), already in clinical use for immunosuppression in transplant patients, were well tolerated and effective in phase I/II cancer trials, and seem an especially promising approach in patients whose tumors lack PTEN.

Targeting distal checkpoints of cell death control

In addition to immunization strategies, targeting IAPs in tumor vaccination protocols, small-molecule IAP antagonists, ASOs targeting IAPs, as well as Smac peptidomimetics are in the process of clinical development or currently in phase I clinical trials, and have been shown to induce and sensitize tumor cells to apoptosis. Murine knockout models confirm the notion that normal cells have fewer drives to caspase activation, and are therefore less dependent on IAPs, thus providing the basis for a therapeutic indication.

Further reading

Ashkenazi A. Targeting death and decoy receptors of the tumor-necrosis factor super-family. Nat Rev Cancer 2002; 2: 420–30.

Cory S, Adams JM. The Bcl2 family: regulators of the cellular life-or-death switch. Nat Rev Cancer 2002; 2: 647–56.

Danial NN, Korsmeyer SJ. Cell death: critical control points. Cell 2004; 116: 205–19.

Ferreira CG, Epping M, Kruyt FA, et al. Apoptosis: target of cancer therapy. Clin Cancer Res 2002; 8: 2024–34.

Fesik SW. Promoting apoptosis as a strategy for cancer drug discovery. Nat Rev Cancer 2005; 5: 876-85 [Erratum: 995].

Ghobrial IM, Witzig TE, Adjei AA. Targeting apoptosis pathways in cancer therapy. CA Cancer J Clin 2005; 55: 178–94.

Gleave ME, Monia BP. Antisense therapy for cancer. Nat Rev Cancer 2005; 5: 468–79.

Greil R, Anether G, Jorer K, Tinhofer I. Tracking death dealing by Fas and TRAIL in lymphatic neoplastic disorders: pathways, targets, and therapeutic tools. J Leukoc Biol 2003; 74: 311–30.

Hu W, Kavanagh JJ. Anticancer therapy targeting the apoptotic pathway. Lancet Oncol 2003; 4: 721–9.

Igney FH, Krammer PH. Death and anti-death: tumour resistance to apoptosis. Nat Rev Cancer 2002; 2: 277–88.

Perona R, Sanchez-Perez I. Control of oncogenesis and cancer therapy resistance. Br J Cancer 2004; 9: 573–7.

Reed JC. Apoptosis-targeted therapies for cancer. Cancer Cell 2003; 3: 17–22.

Rowinsky EK. Targeted induction of apoptosis in cancer management: the emerging role of tumor necrosis factor-related apoptosis-inducing ligand receptor activating agents. J Clin Oncol 2005; 23: 9394–407.

Senderowicz AM. Targeting cell cycle and apoptosis for the treatment of human malignancies. Curr Opin Cell Biol 2004; 16: 670–8.

Shiozaki EN, Shi Y. Caspases, IAPs and Smac/DIABLO: mechanisms from structural biology. Trends Biochem Sci 2004; 29: 486–94.

Tinhofer I, Biedermann R, Krismer M, Crazzolara R, Greil R. A role of TRAIL in killing osteoblasts by myeloma cells. FASEB J 2006; 25 [Epub ahead of print].

Zhivotovsky B, Kroemer G. Apoptosis and genomic instability. Nat Rev Mol Cell Biol 2004; 5: 752–62.

Angiogenesis

J Fayette
Hôpital Edouard-Herriot, Lyon, France

J C Soria
Institut Gustave Roussy, Villejuif, France

Introduction

Cancer cells are dependent on blood vessels for growth and metastases. They cannot survive more than 200 µm away from an existing blood vessel, and tumors rarely exceed 2–3 mm³ without neovascularization. This phenomenon is called angiogenesis and corresponds to the development of new capillaries from existing vessels and the creation of new vessels from circulating endothelial progenitor cells.

Under normal conditions, blood vessels remain quiescent, and angiogenesis occurs only in certain physiological (ovulation, menstrual cycle, pregnancy, and wound healing) or pathological processes (cancer, inflammation, and retinopathy). Numerous factors control angiogenesis. Advances in the understanding of angiogenesis have led to the development of anti-angiogenic therapies (blocking pro-angiogenic or miming anti-angiogenic natural factors) that show efficacy in clinical practice.

Physiopathology

Angiogenesis is finely balanced by pro- and anti-angiogenic factors (Table 8.1). Under normal conditions, the balance leans toward the anti-angiogenic phenotype. Hypoxia is the major element of the angiogenic switch, which leads to overexpression of angiogenic factors, mostly vascular endothelial growth factor (VEGF), favoring new vessel formation. Hypoxia-inducible factor 1α (HIF1α) is naturally expressed and degraded by tumor cells, and under hypoxic conditions, this protein is stabilized and induces several genes, including *VEGF*. The von Hippel–Lindau gene *(VHL)*, which suppresses gene expression induced by hypoxia, is often mutated in cancer. Other determinants of neovascularization are low pH, hypoglycemia, and inflammation with cyclooxygenase-2 (COX2) as well as prostaglandin production.

Table 8.1 Natural modulators of angiogenesis (not an exhaustive list)

Natural inducers of angiogenesis		Natural inhibitors of angiogenesis	
VEGF	Vascular endothelial growth factor	Thrombospondin	
bFGF	Basic fibroblast growth factor	Angiostatin	
aFGF	Acidic fibroblast growth factor	Endostatin	
PDGF	Platelet-derived growth factor	Ang-2	Angiopoietin-2
HGF	Hepatocyte growth factor	IFN-α, IFN-γ	Interferon-α and -γ
EGF	Epidermal growth factor	IL-12	Interleukin-12
TGF-α, TGF-β	Transforming growth factor α and β	Fibronectin	
TNF-α	Tumor necrosis factor α	TIMPs	Tissue inhibitors of metalloproteinase
PGF	Placental growth factor	PAI-1	Plasminogen activator inhibitor 1
Ang-1	Angiopoietin-1	Retinoic acid	
IL-8	Interleukin-8	Dopamine	

The first step in angiogenesis is an increase in vascular permeability, mediated by VEGF, which permits recruitment of growth factors and tissue proteases. This leads to proliferation of endothelial cells and growth of new vessels. These are stabilized by the formation of a new basal membrane and recruitment of mural cells (pericytes for microvessels and smooth muscle cells for larger vessels). Numerous molecular interactions between cells mediate these processes.

Finally, angiogenesis brings nutrients to the tumor cells and allows metastases through fragile and fenestrated vessels.

Growth factors in angiogenesis

Various receptor tyrosine kinases (RTKs) and their ligands act in angiogenesis, particularly the VEGF family and its receptors. The VEGF family comprises 5 members (VEGF-A, … ,-E). The most studied is VEGF-A (simply called VEGF). It is the most powerful stimulator of angiogenesis, inducing proliferation of endothelial cells and preventing their apoptosis. It acts mostly at an early stage of angiogenesis.

Alternative splicing of VEGF leads to five isoforms that are soluble or bound to heparin but have similar efficiency. Three receptors for VEGF are known: VEGFR1, (Flt-1), VEGFR2 (KDR), and VEGFR3 (Flt-4), R3. VEGFR1 and VEGFR2 are expressed on endothelial cells. Hypoxia induces them, and the positive signal is transmitted by VEGFR2, with VEGFR1 possibly acting as a negative regulator. VEGFR3 is expressed by lymphatic endothelial cells and could be responsible for lymph node metastases. A paracrine loop may exist.

Fibroblast growth factor (FGF) and hepatocyte growth factor (HGF) stimulate endothelial cells and the production of VEGF. At a later stage, Ang-1, through its receptor Tie-2, cooperates with VEGF to induce platelet-derived growth factor (PDGF) in endothelial cells. PDGF allows the stabilization of new vessels, recruiting pericytes and smooth muscle cells. This stabilization is crucial, because endothelial cells, which until this stage are dependent on VEGF to prevent their apoptosis, become independent of this factor. Cross-activation characterizes these RTKs, since they can be activated by their natural ligand but also by lymphokines and neurotransmitters.

Anti-angiogenic treatment

Mechanisms of action of anti-angiogenic therapies are many, including destruction of tumor vessels (and thus the killing of a fraction of cancer cells) as well as normalization of the tumor vasculature.

Most approaches targeting the major mediator of angiogenesis, VEGF, alone have been disappointing and have not led to increased survival. However, such approaches combined with chemotherapy in a first-line setting have significantly enhanced survival of patients with colorectal, breast, or lung cancer.

Unlike normal blood vessels, tumor vessels are structurally and functionally abnormal. The presence of aberrant endothelial cells, abnormal pericytes that are loosely attached or absent, and an irregular basement membrane contributes to the formation of poorly organized, dilated, and tortuous blood vessels.

The tumor microenvironment is characterized by interstitial hypertension due to vascular hyperpermeability, and tumor vessels are unable to maintain gradients between vascular and interstitial pressure. This lack of a gradient, with the associated compression of blood vessels by the cancer cells, can impair the flow of fluids, macromolecules, and blood supply. Tumor cells become hypoxic due to the poor oxygen delivery, and hypoxia may cause resistance to both chemotherapy and radiation.

These abnormal characteristics of solid tumors may significantly impair the delivery of therapeutic agents, and it has been shown that anti-angiogenic therapy can normalize the tumor vasculature, thus allowing better delivery of drugs and oxygen to a larger fraction of tumor cells. This concept of normalization may explain the synergy of anti-angiogenic therapy with chemotherapy.

Tumors develop mechanisms of resistance to anti-angiogenic therapies:

- They can overexpress other angiogenic factors or activate other pathways.
- p53 mutations confer resistance to hypoxia, which increases the genetic instability of tumor cells and their proliferation.
- Cancer cells can mimic vessels.
- Endothelial cells may acquire mutations.

Clinical implications

Advances in biology have permitted the characterization of the molecular mechanisms of angiogenesis. VEGF appears to be one of the key players, and therefore current anti-angiogenic strategies have mainly aimed at targeting the VEGF pathway.

The main strategies involve the targeting of:

- VEGF – mainly by monoclonal antibodies or peptibodies
- VEGFR – either by monoclonal antibodies or by broad-spectrum multitarget small tyrosine kinase inhibitors (TKIs) that inhibit phosphorylation in different pathways of angiogenesis signal transduction

The crucial point is the evaluation of treatment:

- In a laboratory setting, angiogenesis is evaluated in the rat cornea, where growth of new vessels can be determined and the efficacy of anti-angiogenic drugs can be observed directly.
- Determination of serum VEGF levels is disappointing, since there is little correlation with either the stage of the disease or the efficacy of treatment.
- Measurement of microvessel density on tumor slides is correlated with angiogenesis activity, but follow-up requires repeat biopsies.
- Circulating endothelial cells could reflect the level of angiogenesis in tumors, and their decrease could be correlated with the efficacy of therapies.
- It is difficult to demonstrate activity according to the Response Evaluation Criteria in Solid Tumors (RECIST) usually employed to evaluate tumor response. Indeed, clinical benefit is observed without a decrease in tumor size on computed tomography (CT) scans. In fact, tumor necrosis may be responsible for an intratumoral edema that can be considered as disease progression although treatment is efficient.
- Dynamic contrast-enhanced magnetic resonance imaging (DCE-MRI) and Doppler ultrasound can help to evaluate the mechanisms of action of anti-angiogenic drugs: intratumoral vascular flows are dramatically and rapidly decreased during the first days of treatment.
- [^{18}F]fluorodeoxyglucose positron emission tomography (FDG-PET) scintigraphy may show a large decrease in the metabolism in tumors.

Clinical use

Several drugs have been tested with success in phase III studies (Table 8.2).

Monoclonal antibodies

- In metastatic colorectal cancer, bevacizumab significantly enhances the response rate (RR) from 34.8% to 44.8% and the median overall survival from 15.6 to 20.3 months when added to an irinotecan/5-fluorouracil (5-FU) combination. The 5-month benefit of bevacizumab is independent of the

Table 8.2 Phase III studies with anti-angiogenic drugs beneficial for overall survival

Type of cancer	Treatment[a]	Objective reponse rate (%)
Colorectal	Irinotecan, 5-FU ± bevacizumab	44.8 vs 34.8 ($p=0.004$)
Colorectal (second-line after irinotecan)	FOLFOX 4 ± (5-FU, FA, oxaliplatin) ± bevacizumab	21.8 vs 9.2 ($p=0.0001$)
Lung (non-squamous, non-small cell)	Paclitaxel/carboplatin ± bevacizumab	27.2 vs 10 ($p=0.004$)
Breast	Paclitaxel ± bevacizumab	28.2 vs 14.2
Renal	Sorafenib	
Gastrointestinal stromal and renal tumors	Sunitinib	

[a] 5-FU, 5-fluorouracil; FA, folinic acid (leucovorin).

chemotherapy, since it is similar with the 5-FU/folinic acid (FA, leucovorin) combination. In the second-line setting, the benefit is lower, and disappears in the third-line setting.

■ In advanced lung adenocarcinoma, first-line bevacizumab in combination with carboplatin/paclitaxel significantly enhances the RR from 10% to 27.2% and the 2-year overall survival rate from 16.9% to 22.1%.

■ In first-line therapy of advanced breast cancer, bevacizumab was added to weekly paclitaxel: the RR increased significantly from 14.2% to 28.2% and the progression-free survival (PFS) from 6.11 to 10.97 months. In second-line treatment, bevacizumab did not result in benefit.

■ These studies also revealed the toxicity profile of bevacizumab (and more generally of all anti-angiogenic therapies): hypertension, thromboembolism, and hemorrhage mostly at the tumor or at proximity of large vessels (there were several toxic deaths in patients with lung cancer).

Oral agents

Broad-spectrum TKIs are active in pretreated cancer patients and in first-line therapy, probably because they inhibit several pathways.

■ Sunitinib inhibits VEGFR1, PDGFR, and C-Kit (the receptor for stem cell factor). In a phase II study, 63 patients with renal cell carcinoma

(RCC) received sunitinib after failure of a cytokine. It resulted in 25 (40%) partial responses (PR) and 17 (27%) stabilizations (SD). In this setting of second-line treatment in RCC, objective response rates are usually just above 5%. The median time to progression in the 63 patients was 8.7 months and the median survival 16.4 months. Based on these results, a phase III trial comparing sunitinib with interferon-α (IFN-α) in untreated RCC patients was undertaken. This phase III trial is positive (RR 31% vs 6%; progression-free survival 11 vs 5 months).

- Sunitinib has also shown clinical activity in gastrointestinal stromal tumors (GIST) in two studies, after failure of imatinib. Ninety-seven patients (92 evaluable) enrolled in a phase II study received sunitinib: 8 (8%) PRs and 68 SDs (70%; 36 of them for more than 6 months) were observed. A phase III trial is also positive.

- Sorafenib is a potent inhibitor of Raf-1, a key enzyme in the Ras/Raf/MEK/ERK signaling pathway, and an inhibitor of VEGFR2 and PDGFR-β involved in angiogenesis. The TARGET phase III trial confirmed the efficacy of sorafenib in 769 patients with RCC who had failed prior treatment. The PFS was 24 weeks in the sorafenib group and 12 weeks in the best supportive care group ($p=0.00001$), although an objective response was observed in only 2% of the patients. Grade 3 or 4 toxicities included a hand–foot skin reaction (5%), diarrhea (1%), fatigue (2%), and hypertension (1%).

- AG 013736 inhibits VEGFR, PDGFR and c-Kit. Antitumor activity was present in 52 patients with metastatic RCC who had failed prior cytokine-based therapy. AG 013736 (5 mg bid) induced a PR in 46% of patients and stable disease in a further 40%.

- PTK/ZK inhibits the tyrosine kinase activity of VEGFR1, VEGFR2, and PDGFR, and is administered orally. PTK/ZK (1250 mg/d) combined with the FOLFOX 4 regimen (5-FU, FA, oxaliplatin) was subsequently compared with a placebo in the CONFIRM-1 phase III trial, in which 1168 patients with untreated metastatic colorectal cancer were randomized. Neutropenia, thrombocytopenia, and neuropathy did not differ between the two groups. There were more cases of grade 3/4 hypertension (21% vs 6%), venous thrombosis (7% vs 4%), and pulmonary embolism (6% vs 1%) in the PTK/ZK arm, but similar grade 3/4 bleeding and arterial thrombosis. A central review failed to document any significant difference.

- ZD6474 is an inhibitor of VEGFR2, VEGFR3, and epidermal growth factor receptor (EGFR, HER1), albeit to a lesser extent. A clinical trial with docetaxel and ZD6474 has been conducted in patients with advanced non-small cell lung cancer who had progressed after first-line platinum-based chemotherapy. In this randomized phase II trial, 137 patients were randomized to 3 arms: docetaxel plus ZD6474 100 mg/day, ZD6474

300 mg/d, or a placebo. Partial results suggest efficacy, with a difference in PFS of 18.8 weeks versus 17 weeks versus 12 weeks.

Various TKIs are currently being tested in several solid tumors. Sorafenib is being investigated in phase III trials in hepatocellular carcinoma and (in combination with carboplatin and paclitaxel) in metastatic melanoma. Phase I–III trials are also ongoing in head and neck, lung, pancreatic, and prostate cancer, as well as in melanoma and sarcoma.

Conclusions

Angiogenesis is a perfect example of translational research, and illustrates how fundamental knowledge of cancer can lead to substantial therapeutic achievements. Indeed, rapid progress has been achieved in the understanding of angiogenesis, including signaling pathways and their regulation. This has enabled the development of numerous potentially interesting agents, many of which are oral drugs. Angiogenesis targeting is now a clinical reality accessible to more and more patients, due to formal approval of agents such as bevacizumab, sorafenib, and sunitinib. Nevertheless, with such treatments, evaluation of tumor response should be reconsidered, and the development of biomarkers is of major interest. The concept of vasculature normalization illustrates that medicine remains at least partially an empirical science and that even simplistic initial hypotheses can lead to the development of efficient drugs.

Cancer cells and tumor-associated host cells: therapeutic implications

I Madani, M Mareel
University Hospital Ghent/Gent, Belgium

Introduction

Malignant tumors consist of cancer cells and tumor-associated host cells. The interaction between the two categories of cells influences invasion and metastasis, as proposed in 1889 by S Paget. He stated that the microenvironment of each organ, the 'soil', influences the survival and growth of the cancer cells, the 'seed'. This 'seed and soil' theory is broadly supported by clinical observations:

■ Although metastasis starts early, it may become apparent many years after removal of the primary tumor (e.g., bone metastasis from breast cancer and liver metastasis from ocular melanoma).
■ An indication of the role of the 'soil' is the fact that metastases tend to affect certain organs rather than others, a phenomenon termed organ specificity of metastasis.

The cancer cell as 'seed'

■ The cancer cell is the 'seed'; inactivation of suppressor genes and activation of promoter genes create aberrant cell populations that attract host cells and initiate the formation of malignant tumors. It is, however, not excluded that the tumor-associated host cells undergo concomitant but independent genomic alterations. Oncogenic changes in the cancer cell compartment might even be secondary to alterations of the host cells, a phenomenon called landscaper defect.
■ Tumor-associated host cell reactions involve:
  – formation of blood and lymph vessels by endothelial cells and pericytes
  – neurogenesis
  – desmoplasia with conversion of fibroblasts into myofibroblasts
  – leukocyte and macrophage infiltration
  – osteolysis through overactivation of osteoclasts
■ Similar host cell reactions also occur in non-tumoral conditions, such as wounds, infections, and inflammatory diseases. Some aspects of these

reactions are tumor-specific, as proposed by H Dvorak, who described malignant tumors as 'wounds that fail to heal'.

Invasion and metastasis are causes of cancer death. Patients die of local invasion in the case of primary brain tumors, of distant metastasis in the case of melanoma and prostate and breast cancer, or of both locoregional spread and distant metastasis in the case of colorectal and bladder cancer. Since tumor-associated host cells contribute to invasion and metastasis, they should be involved in therapy.

Mechanisms of action

Experiments with mice and with cultured cells support the 'seed and soil' theory of cancer metastasis.

- ■ Circumstantial evidence comes from the observation that metastasis changes with the site of injection of the cancer cells. To test the metastatic capacity of defined cell clones in rodents, a distinction is made between 'artificial' metastasis, where cells are injected directly into the arterial or venous circulation, and 'spontaneous' metastasis, where the cells are injected inside tissues to form a primary tumor. It is easy to understand why some cancer cell clones form artificial but not spontaneous metastases, because in the latter test they have to overcome an additional hindrance, namely intravasation. However, some clones fail to form artificial metastases although spontaneous metastasis occurs, indicating that conditioning at the site of injection by interaction with the host is a prerequisite for metastasis.
- ■ Tests of 'spontaneous' metastasis indicate the existence of site specificity. As a rule, the degree of invasion and metastasis is low with tumors that result from paratopic implantation, i.e., at a site that differs from the one from which they are derived. In contrast, orthotopic implantation produces invasive tumors that do metastasize. In experiments by M Pocard, human colon cancer cells injected subcutaneously into nude mice formed well-delineated benign tumors that were cured by surgery. When the same cells were injected into the wall of the cecum, they produced invasive tumors with lymph node metastases that relapsed after surgery and killed the mice.
- ■ In vivo imaging with fluorescence-labeled cells has greatly facilitated metastasis experiments. D Lyden's group showed that tumor-associated host cells are themselves metastatic. The authors used mice whose bone marrow had been eliminated by ionizing irradiation and then reconstituted by labeled cells that could be recognized in the living animal and on histological sections. Two weeks after subcutaneous injection of cancer cells into such reconstituted mice, bone marrow-derived cells (BMDC) were found at the putative

sites of metastasis, namely the lungs. At this site, cancer cells arrived at least 1 week later than the BMDC. Positivity for vascular endothelial growth factor receptor (VEGFR) and for stem cell factor receptor c-Kit permits recognition of these cells in histological sections of the mice, as well as in human cancers. This example demonstrates that host cells not only participate in cancer metastasis but also prepare the 'soil' for the arrival of metastatic cancer cells.

■ Using transgenic mice that failed to express inhibitors of plasminogen activator, JM Foidart demonstrated that migration of blood vessels towards the cancer cells is a prerequisite for invasion. Furthermore, kinetic analysis of histological sections strongly suggests that angiogenesis precedes invasion.

■ Lack of correlation between the invasiveness of cancer cells in animals as compared with in vitro culture has been very instructive about the role of host elements. In experiments by F Martin, PROb colon cancer cells (a cell line derived from a chemically induced tumor), upon subcutaneous injection into syngeneic rats, produced ulcerating tumors that were poorly differentiated and invaded skin and muscle. These invasive cancers were rich in myofibroblasts, which were localized mainly at the front of invasion. PROb cells harvested from routine cell culture, however, failed to invade when confronted with gels of extracellular matrix or with tissue fragments (frequently used substrata for in vitro testing). In contrast, freshly dissociated tumor cell suspensions, containing PROb cells and tumor-associated stromal cells, were invasive in all the in vitro tests.

■ O De Wever has isolated human fibroblasts and myofibroblasts from fresh surgical specimens of normal and cancerous colon, respectively. Admixture of myofibroblasts, but not of fibroblasts, stimulated the invasion of human colon cancer cells into extracellular matrices in vitro within 2 days. In longer co-cultures in vitro (2 weeks instead of 2 days), fibroblasts also stimulated invasion, because they had transformed into myofibroblasts under the influence of the colon cancer cells.

■ Epithelial-to-mesenchymal transition (EMT) refers to gastrulation in embryonic development, where epithelial cells invade through the primitive streak and convert to mesenchymal cells. EMT is a correlate of cancer cell invasion that can easily be screened under the phase contrast microscope in living cultures on solid substrate and thereafter confirmed molecularly through loss of epithelial markers (e.g., E-cadherin) and gain of mesenchymal markers (e.g., vimentin). This method has led to the isolation from conditioned media of pro-invasive secretory factors, such as scatter factor/hepatocyte growth factor (SF/HGF).

Candidate molecules implicated in the crosstalk between cancer cells and tumor-associated host cells and between different types of host cells (Figure 9.1) are searched for in two ways:

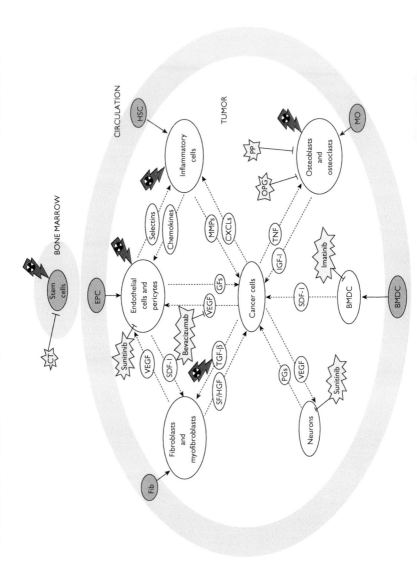

92

Figure 9.1 Schematic representation of tumor-associated host cells and selected examples of their invasion- and metastasis-related molecular crosstalk with cancer cells. Endothelial cells and pericytes build blood and lymph vessels; inflammatory cells comprising lymphocytes, dendritic cells, neutrophils, macrophages, and mast cells pave the way for invading cancer cells; osteoblasts and osteoclasts act at the site of bone metastasis; bone marrow-derived cells prepare sites for metastasis; neurons carry different stimuli causing cancer pain and secrete factors, some of which possess pro-invasive activity; fibroblasts and myofibroblasts establish desmoplastic reaction. Specific markers identify stem cells and precursors in the bone marrow and the circulation: EPC, endothelial precursor cells; HSC, hematopoietic stem cells; MO, monocytes; BMDC, bone marrow-derived cells; Fib, fibrocytes. Dashed lines indicate molecular crosstalk between the cells, exemplified by the folowing: CXCLs, chemokines with a cysteine–other amino acid–cysteine motif; GFs, various growth and invasion factors; IGF-1, insulin-like growth factor 1; MMPs, matrix metalloproteinases; PGs, prostaglandins; SDF-1, stromal cell-derived factor (also called CXCL 2). SF/HGF, scatter factor/hepatocyte growth factor; TGF β, transforming growth factor β; TNF, tumor necrosis factor; VEGF, vascular endothelial growth factor; arrowheads on the dashed lines point to the specific receptors on the cell periphery. Full arrows indicate cellular transition or translocation. Flashes and stars point to putative targets for ionizing radiation and chemotherapy, respectively; bevacizumab is a monoclonal antibody neutralizing VEGF; CT, cytotoxic chemotherapy; sunitinib and imatinib are small-molecule tyrosine kinase inhibitors for the VEGF receptor and c-Kit (stem cell (factor receptor), respectively; OPG, osteoprotegerin, a soluble decoy receptor for RANK (receptor activator of nuclear factor κB (NF-κB)) ligand, a molecule active in signaling from cancer cells to osteoclasts; PP, bisphosphonates

- examination of single molecules (e.g., transforming growth factor (TGF)-β) selected on the basis of their activities in other biological systems
- high-throughput microarray analysis targeting hundreds of genes and their products

Both approaches have led to overwhelming numbers of candidates. M Allinen has published a long lists of genes that are different in tumor-associated host cells in breast cancer as compared with their normal counterparts. Treatment of fibroblasts with TGF-β leads to production not only of SF/HGF but also of hundreds of other proteins. These recent results concerning molecular signaling from tumor-associated host cells add to the complexity of the hundreds of genomic alterations found in cancer cells.

Taken together, there is experimental evidence indicating that various host cells originating locally or in the bone marrow participate in invasion and metastasis. It is striking that these host cells are themselves invasive as they migrate from the local environment into the tumor, and even metastatic as they move from the bone marrow to the tumor. This phenomenon has been called by G Opdenakker 'countercurrent invasion', because cancer cells and host cells take opposite directions, towards the tumor for host cells, away from the tumor for cancer cells. Figure 9.1 schematically presents selected examples of crosstalk between cancer cells and invasion- or metastasis-related host cells, and shows their role as putative targets for therapeutics currently used in the clinic.

Clinical implications

How cancer therapy affects tumor-associated host cells and how this influences invasion and metastasis has hardly been investigated. Given their assistance to invasion and metastasis, these host cells are attractive targets for therapy, especially as they are expected to be sensitive to routine therapeutic agents (Figure 9.1).

The specific reactions of these cells in their tissue context will, however, be complex, as exemplified by ionizing radiation. This is characterized by its rapid (within nanoseconds) molecular signaling, by stimulation of the secretion of cytokines, growth factors, and proteases, by the hormetic nature of its effects (opposite at lower as compared with higher doses), and by the existence of acute and long-lasting late tissue reactions.

Osteoclasts and their monocyte precursors are inhibited by low doses of radiotherapy, as evidenced by the rapid analgesic response of bone metastases.

At low doses, ionizing radiation cures hemangiomas. This anti-angiogenic effect is probably due to induction of apoptosis in endothelial cells.

Ionizing radiation may, however, also stimulate cellular activities serving angiogenesis, as suggested by increased migration and production of matrix-degrading enzymes by endothelial cells in culture. Remarkably, lymphatic vessels in the peritumoral area are more radioresistant than blood vessels, and may safeguard one of the routes for metastasis.

The consequences for invasion and metastasis of radiation-induced alterations in inflammation and immunity are virtually unpredictable, as these alterations come in waves with various types of inflammatory cells and immunocytes that have different radiosensitivity. Most of these cells are easily cleared from sites of inflammation – a fact well known by experienced radiotherapists who routinely treated inflammatory conditions and kidney transplant rejection with low doses of radiation. At the same time, ionizing radiation, producing apoptosis-associated chemokines, may chemoattract from the circulation leukocytes that exert pro-invasive activities. Normal and tumoral stroma, comprising (myo)fibroblasts and extracellular matrix, is regulated mainly by TGF-β. Ionizing radiation stimulates the release of active TGF-β from its latent complex through the production of reactive oxygen species that are generated in low doses immediately after exposure. In the tumor, activated TGF-β mediates a number of cellular activities that are implicated in invasion, namely mesenchymal proliferation with transition of fibroblasts into myofibroblasts, recruitment of inflammatory cells, remodeling of extracellular matrix through production of collagen, and activation of matrix-degrading enzymes. Understandably, fibrosis is the most common late side-effect of radiotherapy. Conversely, ionizing radiation is used to prevent acute postoperative stromal reaction in periarthritis ossificans.

Like radiotherapy, chemotherapy using the first-generation cytotoxic agents as well as newer modulators of signaling pathways acts on host cells as well as on cancer cells.

Clinical use

Understanding the effect of cancer therapy on metastasis-related host cells may lead to modulation of therapeutic strategies both at the primary tumor and at the site of metastasis.

In the view of many clinicians, current forms of cancer treatment change the pattern of metastasis without necessarily altering survival time – an impression that needs to be substantiated. How far is the pattern of metastasis influenced by the response of host cells to therapy? Serendipitous prevention of metastasis has occurred in parts of the skeleton included in radiation fields applied for the treatment of breast cancer. Low doses (approximately 10 Gy) suggest that host cells rather than cancer cells are the target. Intentional prevention of metastasis is achieved by irradiation of the brain in the case of lung cancer and of the lungs in the case of sarcoma. Here, successful prevention can be explained through eradication of the 'seed', namely small deposits of cancer cells (micrometastases), or alteration of the 'soil', namely host cells that participate at the development of metastases. If the 'soil' were taken as the target, lower doses might be considered, with less toxicity.

Conclusions

In summary, we suggest:

- the inclusion of host cells in the evaluation of therapeutic response and patient follow-up
- the extension of indications for radioprevention of metastasis, including dose–response studies

Acknowledgment

The authors thank Professor W De Neve for discussions.

Further reading

Barcellos-Hoff MH. How do tissues respond to damage at the cellular level? The role of cytokines in irradiated tissues. Radiat Res 1998; 150: S109–20.

De Wever O, Mareel M. Role of tissue stroma in cancer cell invasion. J Pathol 2003; 200: 429–47.

Kaplan RN, Riba RD, Zacharoulis S, et al. VEGFR1-positive haematopoietic bone marrow progenitors initiate the pre-metastatic niche. Nature 2005; 438: 820–7.

McBride WH, Chiang CS, Olson JL, et al. A sense of danger from radiation. Radiat Res 2004; 162: 1–19.

Vakaet LAM-L, Boterberg T. Pain control by ionizing radiation of bone metastasis. Int J Dev Biol 2004; 48: 599–606.

New drug development

10

MW Lobbezoo
NDDO Research Foundation, Amsterdam, The Netherlands

E van der Putten
INC Research, Amsterdam, The Netherlands

Introduction

Developing effective anticancer agents with a reasonable safety margin was difficult in the past. Many agents have entered clinical trials in cancer patients, particularly since the 1980s. However, most agents that have been developed since this time have failed at various stages of development due to unacceptable toxicity in preclinical studies or early clinical trials or to lack of efficacy on clinical endpoints, or because the toxicity appeared too difficult to manage in a larger patient population.

With the emergence of targeted anticancer agents in the clinical development arena, it has become necessary to reconsider the way in which anticancer drug development is conducted. Targeted agents have necessitated a re-evaluation of the drug development template used in the development of conventional anticancer chemotherapy in the past.

Anticancer drug development

Historically, anticancer drug therapy using cytotoxic agents has largely been a last resort for cancer patients with metastatic disease. Conventional cytotoxic agents are generally directed at processes of cell division in the cell nucleus. Thus, they affect all dividing cells, not only tumor cells, increasing the likelihood of damage to healthy tissues.

For several types of cancer, no or hardly any effective cytotoxic drug therapy is available (e.g., metastatic melanoma), while the efficacy of drug therapy in other cancers is often limited to reducing or temporarily stopping tumor growth, with limited overall survival benefit (e.g., non-small cell lung cancer and colorectal cancer).

In recent years, targeted anticancer agents have become the focal point in clinical development, and several have entered daily clinical practice. These agents have a well-defined molecular target, usually a molecule that has been demonstrated to play a role in the pathophysiology of cancer (e.g., carcinogenesis, cell cycle regulation, tumor progression and metastasis, tumor angiogenesis, or apoptosis). Many potential target molecules have been identified and are being pursued in clinical trials of agents aimed at affecting specific targets.

Hallmarks of targeted anticancer agents are:

■ modest toxicity, particularly when compared with conventional cytotoxic agents
■ a stabilizing effect on tumor growth rather than induction of tumor regression

Their mild toxicity profile has enabled daily administration of several targeted agents, often by the oral route, rendering long-term continuous therapy a realistic option. Targeted agents are to be viewed as a class that is clearly distinct from conventional anticancer chemotherapy, which is usually so toxic that it can only be given intermittently, with a recovery period after each course of chemotherapy.

Conventional anticancer drug development

The development of anticancer agents is a stepwise process, usually subdivided into relatively distinct phases.

Drug discovery

Chemists and biologists design and discover potential anticancer agents. Large series of chemicals have been screened for antitumor activity, including newly synthesized molecules, analogs of available suboptimal agents, and natural products. Anticancer drug discovery has been hampered significantly by the weak, predictive value of preclinical models for human cancer.

Preclinical development

The main aim of preclinical development is to prepare a drug candidate for first-in-human studies or to stop development if the drug does not meet essential biological/chemical/pharmaceutical requirements. The main issues addressed are:

■ production of the drug substance in sufficient amounts and of adequate quality

- development of a suitable dosage form
- defining the most important pharmacokinetic characteristics in animals
- defining a safe starting dose for the intended route and frequency of administration in subsequent clinical trials
- describing the toxicity profile in animals, focusing on vital functions and target organ toxicity

The latter two are the primary objectives of preclinical toxicology studies, which can often be conducted in rodents only and with short-lasting exposure to the drug.

Phase I clinical studies

Compared with other therapeutic areas, phase I studies of anticancer agents have been very typical because of the high potential for toxicity in man. Phase I studies in oncology are conducted in cancer patients who have no therapeutic options left, rather than in healthy volunteers.

A typical phase I study is a dose escalation study, starting at a presumably safe dose, with dose escalation in a subsequent cohort of patients until dose-limiting toxicities (DLTs) are observed. The dose level at which this occurs is declared the maximum tolerated dose (MTD). A subsequent cohort of patients is then entered at a dose just below the MTD to see whether that dose might be used in subsequent phase II studies.

The preferred route of administration in most conventional phase I studies has been intravenous delivery, as this eliminates the possible impact of variability in drug absorption on the outcome. This requires sufficient solubility and stability of the drug in a vehicle that can be infused.

Phase II clinical studies

Phase II studies are mostly disease-orientated, exploratory studies looking for signs of clinical activity, mostly partial or complete tumor responses according to the Response Evaluation Criteria in Solid Tumors (RECIST) or the World Health Organization (WHO) criteria. The use of a panel of tumor types investigating the objective response rate (ORR: the percentage of patients having a partial or complete tumor response) for each tumor type is an approach that is frequently followed in oncology drug development programs. Such exploratory phase II studies can often be completed with as few as 15–25 patients. If an ORR > 20% is achieved, the tumor type is considered to be sensitive to the drug and a potential indication for confirmatory, more extensive phase II studies and/or pivotal phase III studies, incorporating endpoints such as time to disease progression, overall survival, and quality of life (QoL).

Another important secondary aim in this phase is further exploration of the safety/toxicity of the drug.

Phase III clinical studies

Phase III studies are generally disease-oriented trials to confirm clinical benefit in a given tumor type. These trials are usually designed as comparative studies of the experimental agent, alone or in combination with standard agents, and a standard drug regimen (often a combination of chemotherapeutic agents). A new drug may also be investigated as a replacement for one of the agents in an established combination regimen. If no active standard regimen is available, best supportive care may be an appropriate comparator.

Endpoints frequently used in phase III studies include ORR, progression-free survival, overall survival, and symptom control/QoL.

A typical phase III pivotal study in advanced cancer is powered to demonstrate a few months' survival benefit for the experimental arm, and usually requires several hundred patients.

New anticancer agents have been approved on the basis of better tolerability, improved symptom control/QoL, and/or greater patient convenience (e.g., oral administration versus intravenous infusion).

In cancers where more lines of standard (chemo)therapy are available, a new agent will initially often be tested in the last line of treatment or as the next line after the last current line, as clinicians and ethics committees will be reluctant to deny patients existing standard therapy. Thus, a new anticancer agent will have to work its way forward from later lines of therapy to earlier lines. This may prove difficult in pratice since heavily pre-treated patients entered in studies of later lines of therapy may be generally less susceptible to the benefits of systemic therapy and may be more sensitive to side effects.

Postregistration studies

Once a new anticancer agent has obtained regulatory approval in its first indication, a postregistration clinical trial program may be required to define more precisely the drug's role(s) within the therapeutic armamentarium. Additional indications or earlier lines of therapy in the initial indication may then be investigated. As this may require previously untested combinations with existing agents, additional phase I or II studies may be necessary.

Drug development with targeted anticancer agents

With the emergence of targeted agents in (pre)clinical development, the usefulness of the conventional drug development scheme for anticancer agents is being challenged. Alternative approaches have been proposed and tried. Although this has not yet resulted in one (or more) globally accepted strategy, important points worth consideration have been formulated.

Toxicity profile

The conventional strategy, in particular the phase I/II portion, is largely designed to handle toxic agents. Dose escalation studies aimed at defining DLTs and MTD might seem less than optimal for targeted agents. It has been proposed to introduce biomarkers that are specific to the agent's molecular target and can act as a new type of endpoint in phase I studies to define a biologically relevant dose of the drug and take that dose to phase II/III trials. However, until now, most experts' advice is to determine DLTs and MTD for targeted agents.

The relatively non-toxic nature of most targeted agents implies that such agents could be investigated in phase I studies in healthy volunteers rather than in cancer patients who have exhausted their therapeutic options, provided that certain safety criteria are met (the safety data required for healthy volunteer studies will be more extensive than the current 'minimum safety package' for cytotoxic agents). Data from healthy volunteers may give more reliable information on the biological properties of the agent than results obtained in terminally ill patients. It may also enable the international drug development community to keep up with the increasing demand for phase I capacity for targeted anticancer agents.

Response evaluation

The conventional criterion for selecting an anticancer agent for clinical development has been the drug's ability to induce tumor regression. This approach is invalid for non-cytotoxic agents that are fundamentally unable to induce tumor regression. Other endpoints may be defined, such as the disease control rate (the percentage of patients displaying tumor regression or disease stabilization, as evidenced by a lack of tumor growth over a prolonged treatment period). These new decision-making criteria are needed to determine whether a drug's biological properties warrant its evaluation in larger-scale clinical trials.

Such criteria may have to be drug- or class-specific, as different types of targeted agents may induce different biological effects in the tumor or its environment (e.g., suppressing tumor angiogenesis may be a very relevant biomarker for anti-angiogenic or vascular-targeting agents, but may be irrelevant for agents targeting apoptosis).

Study population

Population enrichment

If the target molecule of a particular targeted agent can be assayed in blood or tissue samples from patients, this may allow the selection of patients who express the specific target (and will therefore be more likely to respond to the targeted agent) and those who do not (or not to a sufficiently large extent).

Study design

Several new study designs are being evaluated to better show activity of targeted agents in cancer patients (e.g., randomized discontinuation trials).

Testing a targeted agent as a single agent in previously untreated (chemotherapy-naive) patients may show the potential benefit of the drug, although this may not be feasible in all tumor types.

Combination with cytoxic agents

Since many targeted agents are merely cytostatic, testing these agents in combination with treatments that are aimed at killing rapidly dividing cells (e.g., cytotoxic anticancer drugs or radiotherapy) seems irrational. However, some targeted agents have been proven to improve the efficacy of anticancer agents (e.g., bevacizumab + irinotecan/5-fluorouracil in colorectal cancer), while in other situations (e.g., gefitinib and chemotherapy in non-small cell lung cancer), no beneficial effect of adding a targeted agent to conventional chemotherapy has been observed.

Thus, adding a targeted agent to a standard cytotoxic chemotherapy regimen should be carefully reconsidered.

Redefining anticancer drug development

In the past, one general template was more or less adequate for the development of the majority of novel anticancer agents. The advent of targeted agents with their broad array of molecular targets and biological effects means that it is unlikely that one single template will prove satisfactory for all new classes of anticancer agents entering clinical development. Anticancer drug development, like drug development in other therapeutic areas, has become much more diversified than it used to be. It seems useful, therefore, to define several new anticancer drug development templates – one for each class of related agents – in order to ensure that experience gained with a drug from that class (e.g., small-molecule signal transduction modulators) will be used to the benefit of the next candidates from the same class.

[This chapter is based on a paper by the authors published in European Pharmaceutical Contractor 2005; 84–90.]

Further reading

Anisimov VN, Ukraintseva SV, Yashin AI. Cancer in rodents: Does it tell us about cancer in humans? Nat Rev Cancer 2005; 5: 807–19.

European Medicines Agency. Note for guidance on evaluation of anticancer medicinal products in man. CPMP/EWP/205/95Rev.3/Corr.

European Medicines Agency. Note for guidance on the pre-clinical evaluation of anticancer medicinal products. CPMP/SWP/997/96.

Floyd E, McShane TM. Development and use of biomarkers in oncology drug development. Toxicol Pathol 2004; 32(Suppl 1): 106–15.

Korn EL, Arbuck SG, Pluda JM, et al. Clinical trial designs for cytostatic agents: Are new approaches needed? J Clin Oncol 2001; 19: 265–72.

Lobbezoo MW, Giaccone G, van Kalken CK. Signal transduction modulators for cancer therapy: From promise to practice? Oncologist 2003; 8: 210–13.

Therasse P, Arbuck SG, Eisenhauer EA, et al. New guidelines to evaluate the response to treatment in solid tumors. J Natl Cancer Inst 2000; 92: 205–16.

World Health Organization. WHO Handbook for Reporting Results of Cancer Treatment. Geneva: WHO Offset Publication 48, 1979.

Inhibition of receptor tyrosine kinases

11

M Bradic, A Östman
Cancer Center Karolinska, Stockholm, Sweden

Tyrosine kinases and cancer

Cell signaling by receptor tyrosine kinases

Tyrosine phosphorylation is a central mechanism for controlling cell signaling leading to proliferation, migration, and differentiation. The enzyme families that control tyrosine phosphorylation are the tyrosine kinases and the protein tyrosine phosphatases. The human genome encodes approximately 90 tyrosine kinases (Figure 11.1). These are further divided into the receptor tyrosine kinases (RTKs) and the cytosolic tyrosine kinases. Most RTKs transmit signals from soluble growth factors, whereas the soluble tyrosine kinases in most cases act as components of intracellular pathways activated by RTKs or other cell surface proteins.

The RTKs contain an extracellular ligand-binding domain, which is connected to the cytoplasmatic intracellular domain by a single transmembrane helix. With the exception of the insulin receptor subfamily, RTKs occur as monomers in the absence of ligand.

Activation of RTKs is now well characterized, and involves multiple steps (Figure 11.2). Activation is triggered by ligand binding to the extracellular domain, which induces dimerization of the receptors. Dimerization leads to autophosphorylation of regulatory tyrosines and kinase activation. The phosphorylated receptor is then able to recruit and activate intracellular signaling enzymes, which initiates signaling events that lead to alteration in gene transcription and ultimately to cellular responses such as proliferation or migration.

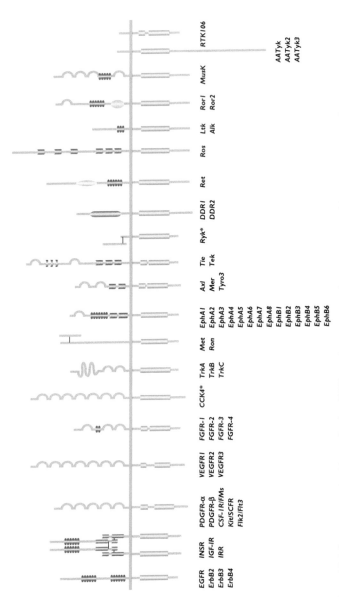

Figure 11.1 Receptor tyrosine kinase families. EGFR, epidermal growth factor receptor; INSR, insulin receptor; IGF-IR, insulin-like growth factor I receptor; IRR, insulin receptor-related receptor; PDGFR, platelet-derived growth factor receptor; CSF-1R, colony-stimulating factor 1 (macrophage colony-stimulating factor) receptor; SCFR, stem cell factor receptor; VEGFR, vascular endothelial growth factor receptor; FGFR, fibroblast growth factor receptor; NGFR, nerve growth factor receptor; HGFR, hepatocyte growth factor receptor. Adapted by permission from Macmillan Publishers Ltd: Nature, Blume-Jensen P, Hunter T. Copyright 2001.

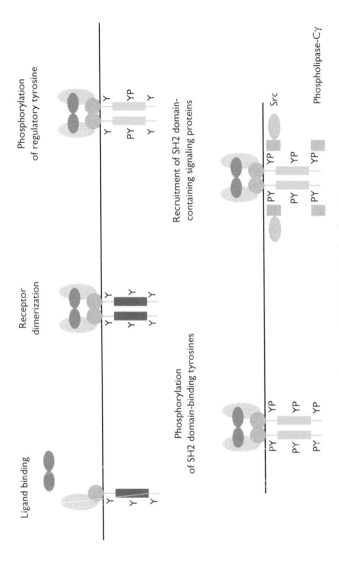

Ligand binding

Receptor dimerization

Phosphorylation of regulatory tyrosine

Phosphorylation of SH2 domain-binding tyrosines

Recruitment of SH2 domain-containing signaling proteins

Src

Phospholipase-Cγ

Figure 11.2 Activation of receptor tyrosine kinase. Y, tyrosine; PY/YP, phosphorylated tyrosine

107

Tyrosine kinases stimulate the growth of malignant cells and tumor stroma

Two key features of solid tumors are:

- the occurrence of malignant epithelial cells characterized by mutational activation of growth-stimulatory pathways
- the presence of genetically stable cells, which make up the supporting tumor stroma that provides, for example, tumor angiogenesis

Tyrosine kinases play critical roles both in the growth of malignant cells and in the formation of tumor stroma.

RTKs involved in driving the growth of malignant cells

Mutational activation of tyrosine kinase activity can occur through chromosomal translocations, gene amplifications, or subtle genetic changes such as point mutations or small deletions. Validated targets for cancer treatment are discussed further below (Figure 11.3).

Activating translocations

Some specific recurrent chromosome translocations give rise to oncogenic tyrosine kinases:

- The t(9;22) translocation (Philadelphia chromosome) in chronic myeloid leukemia (CML) encodes the constitutively active fusion protein Bcr–Abl.
- The t(5;12) translocation creates a gene encoding a ligand-independent variant of the platelet-derived growth factor (PDGF) β-receptor (PDGFR-β) in chronic myelomonocytic leukemia (CMML).

Gene amplification

RTK overactivity can also be caused by gene amplification, which leads to overproduction of RTKs:

- HER2/*neu* (*ERBB2*) may be amplified in breast cancer, and is associated with aggressive clinical behavior. Assessment of HER2 expression status on breast cancer biopsies through immunohistochemistry has therefore widely been incorporated into diagnostic and prognostic routines.

Point mutations and small deletions

Many RTKs become activated by gain of functional mutations caused by point mutations or small deletions. In most cases, these changes affect the kinase domain and lead to enhanced enzymatic activity:

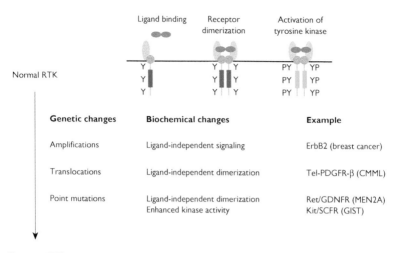

Figure 11.3 *Conversion of receptor tyrosine kinases (RTKs) to oncogenic proteins. PDGFR, platelet-derived growth factor receptor; CMML, chronic myelomonocytic leukemia; GDNFR, glial-derived neurotrophic factor receptor; MEN2A, multiple endocrine neoplasia type 2A; SCFR, stem cell factor receptor; GIST, gastrointestinal stromal tumor*

- c-Kit (the stem cell factor receptor) is activated by mutations in more than 80% of gastrointestinal stromal tumors (GIST).
- The epidermal growth factor receptor (EGFR) has recently been shown to be mutated in a subset of non-small cell lung cancers (NSCLC).

RTKs involved in angiogenesis and in recruitment of tumor fibroblasts

Vascular endothelial growth factor (VEGF) and PDGF receptors are two subfamilies of RTKs that are of special importance for angiogenesis and stroma recruitment:

- VEGFR2 is expressed on normal and tumor endothelial cells, and mediates mitogenic and migratory signals in these cells. The most important ligand for this receptor is VEGF-A.
- VEGFR3 plays a critical role in normal lymphangiogenesis, and has also been implied in the formation of tumor lymphatic vessels.
- PDGFRs are important in the recruitment of pericytes to normal and tumor capillaries. These PDGF-dependent pericytes contribute to angiogenesis

by promoting maturation of newly formed vessels. They are also expressed on tumor fibroblasts and important mediators of stroma recruitment.

Drugs that block VEGFR or PDGFR are now available, and their clinical effects have validated these receptors as highly relevant cancer drug targets.

Drugs inhibiting tyrosine kinase signaling

The term 'targeted therapies' refers to a new generation of cancer drugs designed to interfere with specific proteins that have a critical role in tumor growth and progression.

The inhibitors of tyrosine kinase signaling can be broadly divided into antibodies and low-molecular-weight inhibitors (small molecules) (Figure 11.4):

■ Antibodies:
  – act extracellularly
  – show high specificity
  – act by preventing ligand–receptor interactions by binding either to the ligand or the receptor
  – require intravenous administration
■ Small molecules:
  – bind directly to the intracellular kinase domain
  – act as competitive inhibitors of ATP binding
  – are orally available

Some approved tyrosine kinase inhibitors, and their indication, are presented in Table 11.1.

Inhibitory antibodies

■ Trastuzumab (Herceptin) was the first FDA-approved tyrosine kinase-targeting drug. It is an antibody binding to the extracellular part of HER2. This tyrosine kinase receptor is amplified in approximately 25% of breast cancers. The pivotal study demonstrated significant improved survival by addition of trastuzumab to chemotherapy in HER2-positive metastatic breast cancer. More recently, very encouraging results have been observed when trastuzumab has been used in an adjuvant setting.
■ Bevacizumab (Avastin) works by binding to VEGF-A in a manner that prevents this growth factor from binding to angiogenic VEGFR. The FDA approved bevacizumab in 2004 for the treatment, in combination with chemotherapy, of metastatic colorectal cancer. Recent studies have also

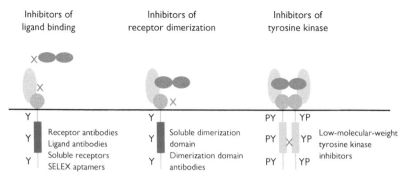

Y	Y	PY | YP
Y	Y	PY | X | YP
Y		PY | YP

Receptor antibodies
Ligand antibodies
Soluble receptors
SELEX aptamers

Soluble dimerization domain
Dimerization domain antibodies

Low-molecular-weight tyrosine kinase inhibitors

Figure 11.4 Mechanisms of action of receptor tyrosine kinase inhibitors

demonstrated a survival benefit of bevacizumab in metastatic breast and lung cancer.

Low-molecular-weight inhibitors of tyrosine kinases

◼ Imatinib (Glivec/Gleevec) was the first member of this category of drugs to be approved based on its activity in CML. Imatinib blocks the kinase activity of the tyrosine kinases Abl, c-Kit and PDGFR-α and -β. Imatinib is now the standard of care for CML, where it acts by blocking the Bcr–Abl protein encoded by the *BCR–ABL* fusion gene of the Philadelphia chromosome. Long-term follow-up studies demonstrated approximately 90% 5-year survival in CML patients on imatinib treatment. This drug is also approved for treatment of GIST, 85% of which are characterized by activating mutations in c-Kit. The successful clinical development of this drug has been achieved by applications in disease types characterized by mutational activation, and strong growth dependency, of imatinib targets.

◼ Erlotinib (Tarceva) is a small molecule that inhibits EGFR. Erlotinib has been approved for treatment of chemoresistant NSCLC. A number of recent studies suggest that this drug is particularly active in a subset of NSCLC patients with activating mutations and/or amplification of EGFR. Ongoing studies are specifically looking at the effects of erlotinib in this patient subset.

◼ Sorafenib (Nexvar) and Sunitinib (Sutent) are representatives of a category of small-molecule drugs sometimes referred to as 'multikinase inhibitors'.

Table 11.1 Examples of tyrosine kinase inhibitors and their indications

Drug	Antibody/ small molecule	Target protein (target cell type)	Indication
Trastuzumab (Herceptin)	Antibody	HER2 (ErbB2) (tumor epithelium)	HER2+ metastatic breast cancer
Imatinib (Glivec/Gleevec)	Small molecule	Bcr–Abl (leukemia cells) c-Kit (tumor epithelium)	Chronic myeloid leukemia GIST
Erlotinib (Tarceva)	Small molecule	EGFR (tumor epithelium)	Chemoresistant lung cancer
Cetuximab (Erbitux)	Antibody	EGFR (tumor epithelium)	Chemoresistant colorectal cancer
Bevacizumab (Avastin)	Antibody	VEGF (endothelial cells)	Metastatic colorectal cancer
Sorafenib (Nexavar)	Small molecule	VEGF (endothelial cells) PDGFR (pericytes) c-Raf (?) (tumor epithelium (?))	Advanced renal cell carcinoma
Sunitinib (Sutent)	Small molecule	VEGFR (endothelial cells) PDGFR (pericytes) c-Kit (tumor cells)	Imatinib-resistant GIST Advanced renal cell carcinoma

EGFR, epidermal growth factor receptor; VEGF(R), vascular endothelial growth factor (receptor); PDGFR, platelet-derived growth factor receptor; GIST, gastrointestinal stromal tumor

These drugs block both VEGFR and PDGFR. This inhibitory profile allows them to exert potent anti-angiogenic activity through simultaneous targeting of endothelial cells and pericytes, which are dependent on VEGFR and PDGFR, respectively. Sorafenib prolongs survival in chemokine-resistant renal cell carcinoma, and induces a prolonged time to progression after first-line treatment with sunitinib. This latter drug is also active in imatinib-resistant GIST by blocking imatinib-resistant variants of c-Kit.

Future perspectives

The introduction of tyrosine kinase inhibitors into clinical practice is a major success of early 21st century oncology. Continued development in this area is likely to occur.

It is predicted that combination therapies with multiple kinase inhibitors will yield better results. These could include combinations designed to interfere with multiple pathways in the malignant cells, as well as combinations aiming to interfere with multiple cell types of solid tumors. It is also expected that an improved 'matching' between proper patient subsets and a particular drug, or combination of drugs, will increase clinical efficacy.

Also, recent findings of activity of second-line inhibitors of Bcr–Abl in CML indicate that resistance to these drugs can be overcome by defining resistance mechanisms.

Finally, the encouraging effects of trastuzumab in an adjuvant setting suggest that the full potential of this drug is best realized in early settings. Results from ongoing studies with other tyrosine kinase inhibitors in adjuvant setting are awaited with optimism.

Obviously, continued work in these areas will be highly dependent on close and well-informed collaboration between oncologists, pathologists, and preclinical researchers. Investment aiming to improve such interactions is therefore highly warranted.

Further reading

Adams GP, Weiner LM. Monoclonal antibody therapy of cancer. Nature Biotechnology 2005; 23: 1147–57.

Blume-Jensen P, Hunter T. Oncogenic kinase signalling. Nature 2001; 411: 355–65.

Klein S, McCormick F, Levitzki A. Killing time for cancer cells. Nature 2005; 5: 573–80.

Sawyers C. Targeted cancer therapy. Nature 2004; 432: 294–97.

Schlessinger J. Cell Signaling by Receptor Tyrosine Kinases. Cell 2000; 103: 211–25.

Shibuya M, Claesson - Welsh L. Signal transduction by VEGF receptors in regulation of angiogenesis and lymphangiogenesis. Experimental Cell Research 2006; 312: 549–60.

Monoclonal antibodies

12

H De Samblanx, D Schrijvers
Ziekenhuisnetwerk Antwerpen–Middelheim, Antwerp, Belgium

Introduction

Tumor cells can express specific antigens that are different or at a higher density than in normal cells, making them possible targets for immunotherapy. These antigens can be used to produce specific monoclonal antibodies (mAbs) that can destroy tumor cells.

The first generation of mAbs was made in immortalized mouse B cells, resulting in a murine protein, and their effect was limited by immunogenicity and a poor ability to recruit immune effector mechanisms. These hurdles were overcome by chimeric and humanized mAbs that contain human constant fragment (Fc) domains and retain targeting specificity by incorporating portions of the murine variable regions. This can be accomplished by grafting either the entire murine variable regions (chimeric antibodies) or the murine complementarity-determining regions (humanization) into the human immunoglobulin G (IgG) framework (Figure 12.1).

Mechanisms of action

mAbs have different effects (Figure 12.2):

- antibody-dependent cellular cytotoxicity (ADCC)
- complement-dependent cytotoxicity (CDC)
- alteration of signal transduction within the tumor cell
- elimination of a critical cell surface antigen

They can also be used to target loads (e.g. radioisotopes, drugs, or toxins) to directly kill tumor cells or to activate prodrugs specifically within the tumor (antibody-directed enzyme prodrug therapy, ADEPT).

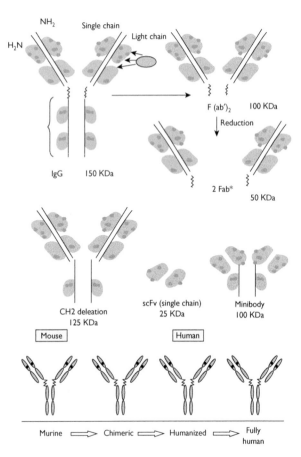

Figure 12.1 Schematic representation of an immunoglobulin G (IgG) antibody, its chemically produced fragments, and several recombinant antibody fragments with their nominal molecular weights. At the bottom, a schematic representation of the process involved in engineering murine monoclonal antibodies (mAbs) to reduce their immunogenicity is provided. A chimeric antibody splices the variable portions (VL and VH) of the murine IgG light chain and heavy chain to a human IgG. A humanized antibody splices only the complementarity-determining region (CDR) portions from the murine mAb, along with some of the adjacent 'framework' regions to help maintain the conformational structure of the CDRs. A fully human IgG can be isolated from specialized transgenic mice bred to produce human IgG after immunizing with tumor antigen or by a specialized phage display method. CL, light-chain constant region; CH1, CH2, CH3, heavy-chain constant regions; NH$_2$, amino terminus; COOH, carboxy terminus

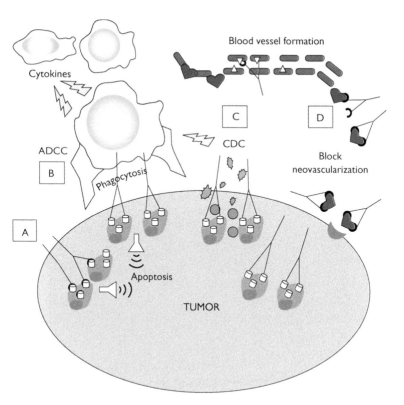

Figure 12.2 Mechanisms of action associated with unconjugated antibodies. In this example, the antigen is shown to be floating in lipid rafts within the tumor cell membrane. (A) Antibodies can activate apoptotic signals by crosslinking antigen, particularly across different lipid rafts. Additional crosslinking of antibody by immune cells can also enhance cellular signaling. (B) Immune cells themselves can attack the antibody-coated cell (e.g., by phagocytosis) and/or they can liberate additional factors, such as cytokines that attract other cytotoxic cells (antibody-dependent cellular cytotoxicity, ADCC). (C) If antibodies are positioned closely together, they can initiate the complement cascade, which can disrupt the membrane, and some of the complement components are also chemoattractants for immune effector cells and stimulate blood flow (complement dependent cytotoxicity, CDC). (D) Tumors also can produce angiogenic factors that initiate neovascularization. Antibodies can neutralize these substances by binding to them, or they can bind directly to unique antigens presented in the new blood vessels, where they could exert similar activities

mAbs can also be used synergistically with traditional chemotherapeutic agents, attacking tumors through complementary mechanisms of action that may include antitumor immune responses.

They can also be associated with radiotherapy to improve the tumoricidal effect of radiation.

Clinical use

mAbs are used in the treatment of hematological malignancies and solid tumors. They are directed toward a wide range of targets:

- cell surface proteins in both solid tumors and individual circulating malignant cells
- antigens associated with the tumoral stroma
- antigens on tumor-associated vasculature
- ligands (e.g., vascular growth factors) that support tumor growth

Epidermal growth factor receptor family

The epidermal growth factor receptor (EGFR) family includes EGFR (also known as c-ErbB1), HER2/*neu* (c-ErbB2), HER3 (c-ErbB3), and HER4 (c-ErbB4).

- HER2/*neu* is overexpressed in 25% of patients with breast cancer and in adenocarcinomas of the ovary, prostate, lung, and gastrointestinal tract. Trastuzumab is a humanized mAb against HER2 that has activity in women with metastatic breast cancer and leads to a reduction in relapse when used in adjuvant setting with chemotherapy in women with HER2-positive breast cancer.
- EGFR is overexpressed in many solid tumors, including non-small cell lung cancer (NSCLC), breast cancer, colorectal cancer, head and neck cancers, and prostate cancer. Cetuximab is a chimeric monoclonal antibody that can induce objective antitumor responses alone or in combination with chemotherapy in patients with cancers overexpressing EGFR. Panitumumab is a humanized mAb with a higher affinity for EGFR than cetuximab. Both of these anti-EGFR mAbs block ligand–receptor interactions. Cetuximab has also been used in combination with radiotherapy and has yielded a superior effect to radiation alone in patients with locally advanced squamous cell carcinoma of the head and neck.

B-cell idiotypes

■ CD52 is a glycopeptide that is highly expressed on T and B lymphocytes. It has been tested as a target for mAbs in the treatment of chronic lymphocytic and promyelocytic leukemias, as well as non-Hodgkin lymphomas (NHL), and as a means to deplete T cells from allogeneic transplant grafts. Alemtuzumab is a humanized anti-CD52 mAb with activity in low-grade NHL.
■ Rituximab is a chimeric anti-CD20 antibody, with activity in CD20+ NHL alone or in combination with chemotherapy.

Vascular endothelial growth factor

Vascular endothelial growth factor (VEGF) and its receptors (VEGFR) have been implicated in promoting solid tumor growth and metastasis by stimulating tumor-associated angiogenesis. Bevacizumab is a humanized mAb that blocks binding of VEGF or VEGF-A to their receptors on the vascular endothelium. Although it has limited activity when given alone, in combination with chemotherapy in patients with previously untreated metastatic colorectal cancer it results in improved objective response rates, median time to cancer progression, and survival compared with chemotherapy alone. Bevacizumab also improves the effect of chemotherapy in patients with metastatic NSCLC and breast cancer.

Toxicity

Monoclonal antibodies are less toxic than cytotoxic chemotherapeutic agents for cancer treatment. However, toxicities do occur, and can be grouped into mechanism-independent and mechanism-dependent categories:

■ Mechanism-independent toxicities relate to the occasional hypersensitivity reactions caused by a protein containing xenogeneic sequences.
■ Mechanism-dependent toxicities result from the binding of a therapeutic antibody to its target antigen:
  – Trastuzumab causes cardiotoxicity because cardiac tissue expresses a small amount of HER2.
  – Rituximab can cause a first-dose toxicity related to the rapid lysis of normal and malignant B cells bearing the target antigen, CD20.
  – Cetuximab causes significant skin eruption based on EGFR expression in skin.
  – Bevacizumab can induce hypertension, bleeding, thrombosis, or proteinuria.

Immunoconjugates have the added toxicities of the conjugated radioactive particles, chemotherapeutic agents, or toxins, including vascular leakage syndrome.

Conclusions

mAbs have a place in the treatment of cancer. However, their cost and side effects may limit their use in clinical practice. The identification of new functional targets and epitopes of existing targets will expand the range of cancers that can be effectively attacked by exploiting mAb technology.

Further reading

Klastersky J. Adverse effects of the humanized antibodies used as cancer therapeutics. Curr Opin Oncol 2006; 18: 316–20.

Sharkey RM, Goldenberg DM. Targeted therapy of cancer: new prospects for antibodies and immunoconjugates. CA Cancer J Clin 2006; 56: 226–43.

Gene therapy

A Vandebroek, D Schrijvers
Ziekenhuisnetwerk Antwerpen–Middelheim, Antwerp,
Belgium

Introduction

Gene therapy encompasses a wide range of treatment types that all use genetic material to modify cells in the treatment of cancer. This may be by insertion of genes into cells or by the use of nucleic acid (either DNA or RNA) to influence protein formation. In theory, it is possible to transform either somatic or germline cells by gene therapy, and gene therapy can be performed ex vivo (modification of cells outside the body) or in vivo (in the body).

Gene therapy can be used to:

- restore mutated genes
- induce activities such as increased immunosuppression
- suppress the expression of certain genes

Vectors for gene therapy

A vector is used to deliver the gene to the target cell.

Viral vectors

The most common vector is a virus that has been genetically altered to carry the information of a human gene. Target cells are infected with the vector, which unloads the genetic material containing the therapeutic human gene into the target cell.

Several viruses have been used to transfer genes into cells:

- Retroviruses have RNA molecules as genetic material. They have reverse transcriptase to translate the RNA into DNA, and integrase to insert this newly formed DNA into host DNA. However, the insertion of this new DNA is uncontrolled and can take place everywhere in the genome. This problem might be overcome by using zinc finger nucleases or by including

121

certain sequences such as the β-globulin locus control region to direct the integration to specific chromosomal sites.

■ Adenoviruses carry their genetic information in double-stranded (ds) DNA. They introduce their DNA into the host, but the genetic material is not incorporated into the host cell's genetic material. The DNA molecule is left free in the nucleus of the host cell, and the instructions in this extra DNA molecule are transcribed like any other gene. However, these genes are not replicated when the cell undergoes cell division and the gene will be lost.

■ Adeno-associated viruses are viruses with single-stranded (ss) DNA. They can insert genetic material at a specific site on chromosome 19. They can carry only a limited amount of DNA.

■ Envelope protein pseudotyping. The envelope proteins of retro- and adenoviruses bind to cell surface molecules. These may be modified to recognize specific epitopes on cells for selective transfection of genes.

Non-viral vectors

Non-viral vectors have the advantage over viruses that they might be produced simply in large quantities and show low host immunogenicity. Their disadvantages are low levels of transfection and expression of the gene compared with viral vectors.

■ Naked DNA is the simplest method of non-viral transfection. However, transfection of cells using this method is relatively low. Naked DNA may be administered by intramuscular injection, electroporation (which uses an external electrical field to increase the permeability of the cell membrane), or a 'gene gun' (which shoots DNA-coated gold particles into the cell using high-pressure gas).

■ Oligodeoxynucleotides are synthetic deoxynucleotides that are used to inactivate genes. They may be used in the following ways:
- Antisense molecules interact with complementary strands of nucleic acids and modify the expression of genes. Antisense nucleic acid molecules bind to mRNA and prevent its translation by degradation of RNA–DNA hybrids by cell nucleases such as RNase H.
- Small interfering RNA (siRNA) may be used to cleave specific unique sequences in the mRNA transcript of a faulty gene, disrupting its translation and expression. Also, siRNAs can be used in the 'triple-helix' strategy, in which inhibitory oligonucleotides (triplex-forming oligonucleotides) target the cellular dsDNA. They interact with polypurine–polypyrimidine sequences in the minor or major groove of genomic DNA and block gene expression at different levels depending on the localization of the complementary sequence.

- Double-stranded oligodeoxynucleotides may act as decoys for transcription factors required to activate the transcription of the target gene. The transcription factors bind to the decoys instead of the promoter of the faulty gene, which reduces the transcription of the target gene, lowering its expression.

■ Lipoplexes and polyplexes facilitate DNA entry into the cell, protecting it from damage. They enter the cell by endocytosis.
- A lipoplex is DNA complexed with lipids. There are three types of lipoplexes: anionic (negatively charged), neutral, and cationic (positively charged). The easiest to use are cationic lipids, which, due to their positive charge, naturally form complexes with the negatively charged DNA and interact with the cell membrane, resulting in endocytosis and release of the DNA into the cytoplasm. Cationic lipids also protect against DNA degradation by the cell.
- A polyplex is a complex of polymers with DNA. Most polyplexes consist of cationic polymers, and their production is regulated by ionic interactions. Unlike lipoplexes, polyplexes cannot release their DNA load into the cytoplasm. Therefore, co-transfection with endosome-lytic agents, which lyse the endosome made during endocytosis (e.g., inactivated adenovirus) is necessary.

Hybrid methods

Every method of gene transfer has its shortcomings. Therefore, some hybrid methods have been developed that combine two or more techniques:

■ Virosomes combine liposomes with an inactivated human immunodeficiency virus (HIV) or influenza virus. They are more efficient for gene transfer in respiratory epithelial cells than either viral or liposomal methods alone.

■ Other viral vectors can be mixed with cationic lipids or hybridizing viruses.

Use of gene therapy

Table 13.1 lists the tumor types in which gene therapy has been tested in early clinical trials.

Tumor suppressor genes

Gene therapy may be used to restore the function of tumor suppressor genes, resulting in control of the cell cycle. Under experimental conditions, it has been demonstrated that restoration of tumor suppressor genes can revert the malignant phenotype.

Table 13.1 Clinical trials of gene transfer for cancer treatment

Gene therapy strategy	Cancer
Drug sensitivity or suicide gene therapy	Mesothelioma
	Brain tumors
	Ovarian cancer
	Colon cancer
	Malignant melanoma
	Breast cancer
	Bladder cancer
	Non-Hodgkin lymphoma
Tumor suppressor gene/oncogene inactivation	Acute myeloid leukemia
	Head and neck cancer
	Colorectal cancer
	Hepatocellular cancer
	Breast cancer
	Ovarian cancer
	Lung cancer
	Prostate cancer
Immunogene therapy	Ovarian cancer
	Brain cancer
	Malignant melanoma
	Prostate cancer
	Colorectal cancer
	Renal cancer
	Head and neck cancer
	Lung cancer
	Breast cancer

■ Transfer of the *TP53 (p53)* tumor suppressor gene has been shown to influence cancer. Several clinical trials based on delivery of wild-type *TP53* using different vectors have observed variable results in different cancer types such as lung, head and neck, bladder, ovarian, and breast cancer.
  – The vector in the first generation of trials was an adenovirus expressing the *TP53* cDNA under the control of a cytomegalovirus (CMV)

promoter, and was used in the treatment of head and neck squamous cell carcinoma

- Another adenovirus vector used the fusion of *TP53* with *VP22*, encoding a tegument protein from herpes simplex virus 1 (HSV-1). The VP22 protein is exported from the cytoplasm of the expressing cell and is incorporated by neighboring cells by poorly defined mechanisms. The fusion of VP22 with other polypeptides enables the intercellular spread of the chimeric protein.

Oncogenes

The aim of gene therapy directed against oncogenes is correction of the imbalance between positive and negative proliferative signals by inhibiting the function of genes involved in the maintenance of unrestricted cell proliferation and acquisition of a metastatic phenotype.

Targets that are being investigated are inhibition of the *RAS* oncogene, *PTTG1* ('pituitary tumor transforming gene 1') and the catalytic subunit of *TERT* ('telomerase reverse transcriptase').

Methods used to inhibit expression of oncogenes are:

- ■ transfer of antisense nucleotides by short sequences (antisense oligonucleotides), or full cDNA
- ■ siRNA
- ■ expression of secreted or intracellular antibody-based molecules that block the function of oncogenes

Gene-directed enzyme or prodrug therapy

Gene-directed enzyme or prodrug therapy (GDEPT) is based on the transfer of exogenous genes that convert a non-toxic prodrug into a cytotoxic metabolite in cancer cells. Once the prodrug has been administered systemically, cells expressing the converting enzyme die and may provoke the destruction of surrounding cells (bystander effect). The efficacy of a GDEPT system is strongly influenced by the extent of the bystander effect, because the fraction of transduced cells in a tumor is generally low with current gene therapy vectors.

- ■ The thymidine kinase gene from HSV-1 (HSV-TK) in conjunction with the prodrug ganciclovir was the earliest and most used GDEPT system. HSV-TK converts ganciclovir into a monophosphate intermediate that is subsequently transformed into the triphosphate form by cellular enzymes. This highly polar molecule cannot diffuse outside the cell and is incorporated into the DNA, causing apoptosis in a cell cycle-dependent manner.

- Yeast cytosine deaminase converts the antifungal drug 5-fluorocytosine into 5-fluorouracil. This metabolite can diffuse locally and cause a wider bystander effect than phosphorylated ganciclovir. Cytotoxicity is cell cycle-dependent.
- Other GDEPT approaches generate very potent DNA crosslinking agents whose effects are largely cell cycle-independent. These include the cytochrome P450/cyclophosphamide and the nitroreductase/dinitrobenzamide systems.
- Delivery of the sodium/iodide symporter (NIS) gene to cancer cells may be used for the internalization of iodine-131. A higher dose is accumulated in cells expressing *NIS*, resulting in cell cycle blockade and cell death.

Expression of cytotoxic or pro-apoptotic genes

It is possible to selectively transfer genes that will cause the destruction of cancer cells by specific mechanisms without any dependence on exogenous drugs. This system relies mostly on the targeting of gene transfer and expression into cancer cells, using specific surface ligands or promoters such as tumor necrosis factor (TNF)-related apoptosis-inducing ligand (TRAIL).

Immunogene therapy

Transfer of genes with the aim of eliciting an immune response against tumor cells is another strategy. Since cancer cells modify their characteristics and their environment to avoid being detected and rejected, an immune response may be triggered by specific gene therapies (immunogene therapies):

- *Expression of immunomodulatory cytokines.* Cytokines, including interleukin (IL)-2, IL-7, IL-12, IL-15, IL-18, IL-21, IL-23, IL-24, interferon (IFN)-α, IFN-β, IFN-γ, TNF-α, granulocyte–macrophage colony-stimulating factor (GM-CSF), and others, are key mediators in the function of the immune system. The use of gene therapy vectors enables localization of cytokine expression in tumor cells, making them more recognizable to the immune system.
- *Vaccination with tumor antigens and genetically modified cells.* The transfer of genes encoding tumor-specific antigens may be used to decrease immune tolerance. Another approach is the administration of activated effector or antigen-loaded presenting cells. The efficacy of these cells can be increased if they are manipulated genetically to express antigens, cytokines or co-stimulatory molecules (ex vivo gene therapy). Also, autologous dendritic cells, which are professional antigen-presenting cells, that express the co-stimulatory molecules (e.g., CD80 or MHC class I and II) may be used for effective activation of effector cells.

Problems

For the safety of gene therapy, it is essential that the gene manipulation of somatic cells is not transmitted to germline cells, influencing offspring.

Other problems of gene therapy include the following:

■ *The short-lived nature of gene therapy*. The therapeutic gene introduced into target cells must remain functional and the cells containing the therapeutic gene must be long-lived and stable. Problems with integrating therapeutic genes into the genome and the rapidly dividing nature of many cells prevent gene therapy from achieving any long-term benefits. Patients may have to undergo multiple rounds of gene therapy.
■ *Immune response*. There is a risk of stimulating the immune system so that the effectiveness of gene therapy decreases. Furthermore, the immune system's enhanced response to vectors such as viruses makes it difficult for gene therapy to be repeated.
■ *Problems with viral vectors*. Viruses present a variety of potential problems to the patient, such as toxicity, immune and inflammatory responses, gene control, and targeting issues. Viral vectors may also cause disease.
■ *Multigene disorders*. A cancer arising from mutations in a single gene is the best candidate for gene therapy. Unfortunately, most cancers are caused by the combined effects of variations in many genes. Multigene or multifactorial disorders such as these would be especially difficult to treat effectively using gene therapy.
■ *Carcinogenesis*. If a gene is integrated in the wrong place in the genome, such as in a tumor suppressor gene, it could induce a tumor.

Conclusions

Gene therapy may be used in the treatment of cancer to directly interfere with cancer genes (tumor suppressor genes or oncogenes) or used to make cancer cells more sensitive to anticancer treatments or the immune system. At present, its clinical use is limited, but some randomized large trials have started.

Further reading

Cross D, Burmester JK. Gene therapy for cancer treatment: past, present and future. Clin Med Res 2006; 4: 218–27.

Cancer vaccines

M Palma, H Mellstedt, A Choudhury
Karolinska University Hospital, Stockholm, Sweden

Introduction

Specific, active immunotherapy (vaccination) for cancer aims at generating or enhancing the immune response to cancer cells. The rationale of this approach is based on the possibility of exploiting the specificity of the immune system to target cancer cells, with little or no associated toxicity to normal cells. Most tumors express tumor-associated antigens (TAA). These are either proteins usually expressed at certain stages of differentiation or only by certain differentiation lineages (e.g., α-fetoprotein (AFP) and carcinoembryonic antigen (CEA)) or proteins expressed at low levels in normal cells and at higher levels in cancer cells, such as growth factors, growth factor receptors, and proteins encoded by oncogenes.

A spontaneous immune response against the TAA, and so against cancer cells, does not occur always or, at least, not to such an extent that it counteracts and stops cancer proliferation. The reason for this is that tumor cells have evolved different mechanisms to evade immune surveillance, which encompass systemic immunological factors as well as the local tumor microenvironment. To have an immune response against TAA, which in most cases are self-antigens, it is also essential that the immune response is shifted from tolerance to immunity. The goal of a successful vaccine is to induce potent tumor-specific immunity and long-lasting immunological memory. This can be achieved by directing the cellular arm of the immune system towards the recognition of TAA, breaking self-tolerance and side-stepping tumor escape mechanisms.

Basic science

Most cancer vaccine strategies investigated up to now have focused on the induction of tumor-specific cytotoxic T lymphocytes (CTL). The combined action of CTL and interferon-γ (IFN-γ)-secreting CD4$^+$ T cells, in fact, is thought to be the most effective immune response to eradicate tumors in

129

vivo. Tumor-specific CD4$^+$ T cells are also critical to mediate the antitumor effector functions of macrophages, eosinophils, and natural killer (NK) cells.

- ■ To initiate an immune response, the antigen must be presented in the context of a major histocompatibility complex (MHC) molecule and in the presence of the appropriate co-stimulatory signals. Tumor cells do not usually express co-stimulatory molecules and are ineffective in priming a T-cell response. The presentation of tumor antigens thus requires the intervention of professional antigen-presenting cells (APC), such as dendritic cells (DC).
- ■ DC are able to stimulate both the innate and the adaptive immune system and to interact with CD4$^+$, CD8$^+$, and NK cells. They present exogenous antigens complexed with MHC class II molecules to helper T cells (CD4$^+$) and endogenous antigens complexed with MHC class I molecules to cytotoxic T cells (CD8$^+$). In this way, CTL are able to detect all the proteins that undergo proteosomal degradation and are presented in the context of MHC class I molecules, encompassing both TAA expressed on the surface of the cancer cell and abnormal proteins synthesized by the cancer cell.
- ■ DC are also able to present exogenous antigens complexed with MHC class I molecules to cytotoxic T cells (cross-presentation and cross-priming).
- ■ Once activated by DC, tumor-specific CTL can kill tumor cells directly. TAA can therefore be used as targets for CTL-mediated killing of tumor cells.

Mechanism of action

Tumor antigens

To prime a CD8$^+$ T-cell response, many different approaches can be effective. Figure 14.1 is a schematic diagram on the various approaches that may be used to deliver tumor antigens for recognition by the immune system:

Tumor cells

- ■ Whole tumor cells, either autologous or allogeneic, can be administered after having been irradiated.
- ■ Allogeneic tumor cell lines can be also used.
- ■ Moreover, to enhance the differentiation and activation of the patient's APC, tumor cells can be genetically engineered to secrete proteins, such as granulocyte–macrophage colony-stimulating factor (GM-CSF), that promote the activation of the APC.

Peptides

- ■ Tumor-derived peptides can be quite easily manufactured and delivered to patients, but carry a human leukocyte antigen (HLA) restriction, which limits their use to patients with a particular haplotype. Tumor-derived

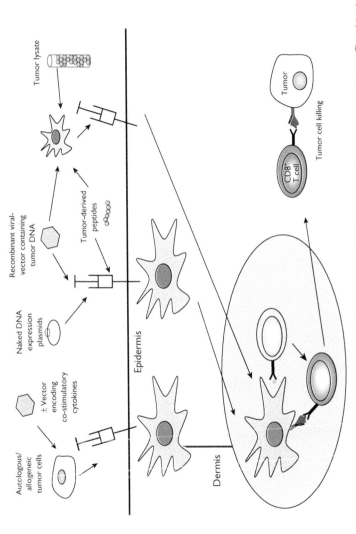

Figure 14.1 Different approaches for delivering tumor-associated antigens (TAA) as vaccines for cancer immunotherapy. The objective of vaccination against cancer is to deliver the TAA in an immunogenic form such that it will be processed and presented to antigen-presenting cells such as dendritic cells (DC) for stimulating antitumor T cells

peptides can also be combined with immunostimulatory molecules to produce a recombinant protein vaccine.

■ Immunization with a whole protein allows multiple epitopes to be presented to CD4+ and CD8+ T cells, and is thus applicable to all patients, regardless of their HLA haplotype.

■ The amino acid sequence of the epitope can be modified to make the vaccination more successful, by increasing its affinity for MHC molecules or T-cell receptor (TCR) triggering or by inhibiting its proteolysis (epitope enhancement). To carry out antigen presentation by APC, then, DC can be expanded in vitro by culturing them from peripheral blood precursors in the presence of GM-CSF, interleukin-4 (IL-4), and tumor necrosis factor α (TNF-α) and then pulsing them either with peptides derived from the TAA or with tumor-derived apoptotic bodies or tumor cell lysate. DC can also be fused with tumor cells or transfected with tumor-derived DNA or RNA.

DNA

■ DNA vaccines are an attractive strategy, providing DC with tumor antigen genes to be processed and presented to CTL. A DNA sequence derived from the TAA can be inserted into a recombinant viral vector that is unable to replicate in the host. This approach has the potential to induce a potent immune response, but also carries the risks of competition with the viral vector epitopes and of possible resistance due to prior systemic immunity to the viral vector.

■ The use of naked DNA expression plasmids, on the other hand, avoids all the problems due to the presence of a viral vector, but induces weaker immune responses.

A summary of the advantages and disadvantages of the different vaccination strategies investigated in clinical trials is provided in Table 14.1.

Adjuvants

■ Immunological adjuvants are substances administered with the vaccine to potentiate the immune response. These can be either chemicals, such as aluminum salts (alum) and incomplete Freund's adjuvant (IFA), or products of microorganisms, such as bacillus Calmette–Guérin (BCG) and lipopolysaccharide (LPS), or recombinant cytokines, such as GM-CSF. With the exception of IFA, whose toxicity profile is not optimal, all these adjuvants have been used in clinical trials and proved to be safe.

■ Their mechanisms of action range from the recruitment of professional APC and/or effector cells (cytokine adjuvants) to acting as a depot for the vaccine (alum) or promoting the secretion of cytokines and/or DC maturation (chemical adjuvants).

Table 14.1 Advantages and disadvantages of different vaccination strategies

Vaccine	Advantages	Disadvantages
Whole tumor cells	• Can be processed to enhance antigen presentation • All relevant TAA virtually expressed • Antigens do not need to be defined	• Require availability of autologous tumor or allogenic cell line sharing the relevant TAA
Gene-modified tumor cells	• Same as whole tumor cells • Can be engineered to coexpress immunostimulatory molecules	• Same as whole tumor cells • Need for ex vivo cell culture • Cost, time, and are labor-intensive
Peptides	• Epitope enhancement possible • Easy to produce and stable • Different peptides can be combined together and/or with immunostimulatory molecules	• Knowledge of the specific epitope needed • HLA restriction
Dendritic cells (DC)	• Powerful APC • Large-scale production of clinical grade DC feasible • Can be loaded with relevant TAA in many ways (e.g., pulsed with tumor-derived peptides or whole proteins, tumor cell lysate; transfected with tumor-derived DNA or RNA)	• Need for ex vivo cell culture • Cost, time, and are labor-intensive • Optimal technique for antigen loading still to be defined • Criteria for standardization of final product still to be defined

TAA, tumor-associated antigen; APC, antigen-presenting cells; HLA, human leukocyte antigen.

133

Combination therapy

The combination of chemo- and immunotherapy can potentially produce a synergistic effect. Chemotherapy could, in fact, enhance the magnitude and duration of the immune response generated by the vaccine by achieving a tumor reduction and provide the optimum immunological milieu, for example by depletion of $CD4^+$ $CD25^+$ regulatory T cells (T_{reg} cells).

Clinical implications

To date, a remarkable number of preclinical and clinical studies have been performed. Overall, vaccine therapy against cancer has proven to have very low associated toxicity. Systemic reactions are generally rare, and adverse effects are normally limited to local reactions, transient mild fever, and erythema.

The vaccine-associated risk of acute or chronic autoimmune reactions is minimal.

In general, however, documented clinical responses with vaccine therapy have been rare, even if some clinical effects have been seen in B-cell malignancies, lung, prostate, and colorectal cancers, and melanoma. Immune responses and clinical responses have often been found to be discrepant, which highlights the necessity for optimization of the design of clinical trials. In this regard, patient selection may be a critical factor.

Clinical use

With their high quality-of-life index and low associated toxicity, anticancer vaccines can today be considered suitable for aged or debilitated patients, otherwise ineligible for more intensive chemo/radiotherapy regimens, but, based on the data available at present, no major and reproducible efficacy is to be expected in most cases. Over the next 10 years, the results of ongoing phase III trials as well as novel immunological adjuvants and better criteria for patient selection will hopefully improve the therapeutic outcome of vaccine therapy, so that this therapeutic modality will become an established form of targeted therapy to be integrated into the standard care of cancer patients.

Further reading

Berzovsky JA, Terabe M, Oh SK et al. Progress on new vaccine strategies for the immunotherapy and prevention of cancer. J Clin Invest 2004; 113: 1515–25.

Gilboa E. The promise of cancer vaccines. Nat Rev Cancer 2004; 4: 401–11.

Combination treatment

BC Kuenen, G Giaccone
Vrije Universiteit Medical Center, Amsterdam,
The Netherlands

Introduction

The treatment of cancer has changed dramatically in the last few years. Until a few years ago, primarily classical chemotherapy was available, represented mainly by drugs that interfere with DNA metabolism and proliferation. With the introduction of targeted therapy, employing compounds directed at dysregulated growth, a new era in the treatment of cancer has begun. These new compounds can be highly effective as single agents in some diseases:

■ Imatinib, a tyrosine kinase inhibitor (TKI) of the Bcr–Abl fusion protein, platelet-derived growth factor receptor (PDGFR), and c-Kit, is highly effective in the treatment of chronic myeloid leukemia (CML) and gastrointestinal stromal tumors (GIST), because it blocks the respective dominant driving forces of malignant cell proliferation in both tumor types.

However, most common solid tumors have multiple genes and gene products that contribute to their malignant behavior, which results in modest therapeutic effects of compounds targeting only one gene product or one pathway:

■ Inhibition of the epidermal growth factor receptor (EGFR) with TKIs in patients with advanced non-small cell lung cancer (NSCLC) results in response rates of only approximately 10% of unselected patients.

For tumors that are heterogeneous, such as most common solid tumors, it is becoming imperative to try to identify the patients who will benefit from targeted therapies. This requires a large effort that includes translational research studies.

Although a few malignancies can be treated successfully with single agents, the greatest gain in the treatment of cancer is probably to be expected from combinations of classical chemotherapy with targeted therapy, combinations of different targeted compounds, and combinations with radiotherapy. The combination of different treatment modalities is appealing, as it has the potential to increase efficacy; this is particularly so when different mechanisms of action are used and when non-overlapping toxicities are observed. The last few years have seen a tremendous number of novel compounds coming to the clinic, and the development of rational combinations has become a major issue.

Design of new combinations and trials should be based on preclinical data and, of course, on clinical experience.

Development of combination treatment

Some examples of the development of combination treatments are discussed here.

Non-small cell lung cancer

Four trials (INTACT-1 and -2, TALENT, and TRIBUTE) failed to show increased efficacy of the addition of gefitinib or erlotinib, two EGFR TKIs, to two different platinum-based doublet chemotherapy regimens as first-line treatment in patients with advanced NSCLC. In all four studies, the EGFR TKI alone was continued after completion of chemotherapy, up until progression or intolerance. Although the studies were negative for the whole population of unselected patients, in the gefitinib arms of the INTACT-2 trial a trend toward improved survival was observed in the subset of patients with adenocarcinoma who had received at least four cycles of chemotherapy. In addition, in the TRIBUTE trial, the subgroup of never-smokers treated with the combination experienced an improvement in survival.

This finding is in line with results obtained with erlotinib and gefitinib as single agents. The biological role of EGFR in NSCLC and additive effects of the combination with several chemotherapeutic agents in preclinical models were the main reasons to combine EGFR inhibitors with chemotherapy. Although no conclusive explanation can be given for the disappointing results of these four trials, which included over 4000 patients, data generated after these large studies point to the lack of patient selection as a major cause.

Although there is no good correlation between response to EGFR inhibitors and level of EGFR expression, mutation status and gene copy number are important predictors of both response and survival outcomes. Patient selection based on clinical characteristics (female, adenocarcinoma, never-smoker) only may be less precise than biological markers. These findings stress the importance of obtaining adequate tumor samples (possibly histological material) and selecting based on standardized validated tests. The results of the four large randomized studies once more raise questions about the validity of preclinical models, especially for combined treatments.

Colorectal cancer

Recent results obtained with targeted compounds added to standard chemotherapy in patients with metastatic colorectal cancer (mCRC) represent good examples of success of combination treatment.

■ A significant improvement in response rate (22.9% vs 10.8%) and median time to progression (4.1 vs 1.5 months) was obtained with the combination of irinotecan plus cetuximab versus cetuximab alone in irinotecan-refractory mCRC patients in a large randomized phase II trial. Cetuximab is a monoclonal antibody against EGFR, and patients for these studies have been selected on the base of being EGFR-positive by immunohistochemistry, unlike the studies performed with EGFR TKIs. It appears logical that only tumors that express EGFR may respond to an antibody that has to bind to the extracellular domain of the receptor; however, recent evidence has shown that EGFR-negative tumors also respond to anti-EGFR monoclonal antibodies. Although data are still limited, patients with tumors with *EGFR* gene amplification (tested by fluorescence in situ hybridization, FISH) experience most benefit from treatment with monoclonal antibodies directed at EGFR. Furthermore, patients with *KRAS* mutations do not appear to benefit from this treatment, in analogy with what was observed in NSCLC treated with EGFR TKIs.

■ Another successful approach of combining chemotherapy and a targeted agent is the introduction of the anti-angiogenic agent bevacizumab in mCRC. Bevacizumab is a monoclonal antibody directed at vascular endothelial growth factor (VEGF). In a randomized phase II trial, 104 patients were randomly assigned to the standard arm 5-fluorouracil/leucovorin (folinic acid) (5-FU/LV) ($500\,mg/m^2$ weekly for 6 weeks of each 8-week cycle), or 5-FU/LV plus high-dose bevacizumab ($10\,mg/kg$ every 2 weeks), or 5-FU/LV plus low-dose bevacizumab ($5\,mg/kg$ every 2 weeks). Although the three treatment arms were not equally balanced, both bevacizumab arms resulted in higher response rates, longer median time to disease progression, and longer survival as compared with FU/LV alone. Because of these observations, a large phase III study was performed, in which more than 800 patients were randomly assigned to receive 5-FU/LV plus bevacizumab ($5\,mg/kg$ every 2 weeks), irinotecan/5-FU/leucovorin (IFL: respectively $125\,mg/m^2$, $500\,mg/m^2$, $20\,mg/m^2$

given 4 out of 6 weeks) plus placebo, or IFL plus bevacizumab 5 mg/kg every 2 weeks. After randomization of 313 patients, interim analysis confirmed the safety of adding bevacizumab to IFL, and therefore the 5-FU/LV arm was discontinued. A significant increase in median overall survival (20.3 vs 15.6 months), progression-free survival (10.6 vs 6.2 months), and response rate (44.8% vs 34.8%) was observed in the combination arm as compared with bolus IFL chemotherapy alone. Besides hypertension (22% all grades and 11% grade 3), toxicity was not increased in the combination arm. Although preclinical models predicted the additive effect of chemotherapy with bevacizumab, the mechanism of interaction is still a matter for speculation; furthermore, the effect of bevacizumab as a single agent is still not fully explored. In this study, no patient selection was performed. Given the pivotal biological role of VEGF in angiogenesis and tumor development, it may be expected that the level of tumor-associated VEGF expression, microvessel density (MVD), or the expression of endogenous anti-angiogenic proteins such as thrombospondin (THBS-1 and -2) would correlate with response to bevacizumab treatment. A retrospective analysis of a representative subset of 312 tissue samples (285 primaries and 27 metastases; 153 from the bevacizumab arm and 125 from the placebo arm) of the large phase III trial has been performed. Epithelial and stromal VEGF expression, stromal THBS-2 expression, and MVD were determined. None of these markers proved to be a significant prognostic or predictive marker, and this study failed to identify a subset of patients more likely to benefit from the addition of bevacizumab to chemotherapy. Given the potential widespread use of bevacizumab in other disease types, it is imperative that further studies be performed attempting to identify the patients that benefit from this approach.

Conclusions

Combination of classical chemotherapy plus targeted therapy is an emerging strategy in clinical oncology, and has become a standard treatment in daily practice for many tumor types. There are, however, numerous challenges to explore and solve. Among these are the selection from a variety of agents that have similar effects, sequences of application, combinations of drugs, individualization and optimization of therapy for a given patient, and identification of patients at risk for important side-effects.

Another interesting observation with regard to combining antiproliferative agents, such as chemotherapy, with eminently cytostatic agents, such as EGFR inhibitors, is that there is a potential negative interaction between these agents, in that the reduction in the number of cells actively proliferating induced by the EGFR inhibitors may negatively influence the effect of chemotherapy. This raises the possible advantage of sequential scheduling of these different treatment modalities. Studies are ongoing that address the issue of scheduling.

In recent years, as a result of many randomized studies performed in unselected patient populations, randomized phase III studies are now more often preceded by relatively small randomized phase II studies, in order to assess feasibility and obtain a rough impression of the potential benefit to be gained from adding the new compound to chemotherapy. This strategy allows a decision to continue into randomized phase III studies to be made with more confidence, compared with a single-arm phase II study, where uncontrolled selection may occur.

Translational research – from bench to bedside and vice versa – should focus on a better understanding of the relation between outcome and the signaling pathways driving tumors, the mechanisms of action of targeted therapy, synergisms among different compounds, the relation between expression of genes and proteins, and the mutational status of genes, in order to improve the results of treatment and to prevent the development of resistance. The development of better and more predictive preclinical models should also be pursued in the quest for a better therapeutic index in patients.

Further reading

Cappuzzo F, Hirsch FR, Rossi E, et al. Epidermal growth factor receptor gene and protein and gefitinib sensitivity in non-small-cell lung cancer. J Natl Cancer Inst 2005; 97: 643–55.

Chung KY, Shia J, Kemeny NE, et al. Cetuximab shows activity in colorectal cancer patients with tumors that do not express the epidermal growth factor receptor by immunohistochemistry. J Clin Oncol 2005; 23: 1803–10.

Cunningham D, Humblet Y, Siena S, et al. Cetuximab monotherapy and cetuximab plus irinotecan in irinotecan-refractory metastatic colorectal cancer. N Engl J Med 2004; 351: 337–45.

Giaccone G. Epidermal growth factor receptor inhibitors in the treatment of non-small-cell lung cancer. J Clin Oncol 2005; 23: 3235–42.

Hurwitz H, Fehrenbacher L, Novotny W, et al. Bevacizumab plus irinotecan, fluorouracil, and leucovorin for metastatic colorectal cancer. N Engl J Med 2004; 350: 2335–42.

Jubb AM, Hurwitz HI, Bai W, et al. Impact of vascular endothelial growth factor-A expression, thrombospondin-2 expression, and microvessel density on the treatment effect of bevacizumab in metastatic colorectal cancer. J Clin Oncol 2006; 24: 217–27.

Kabbinavar F, Hurwitz HI, Fehrenbacher L, et al. Phase II, randomized trial comparing bevacizumab plus fluorouracil (FU)/leucovorin (LV) with FU/LV alone in patients with metastatic colorectal cancer. J Clin Oncol 2003; 21: 60–5.

Lievre A, Bachet JB, Le CD, et al. *KRAS* mutation status is predictive of response to cetuximab therapy in colorectal cancer. Cancer Res 2006; 66: 3992–5.

Moroni M, Veronese S, Benvenuti S, et al. Gene copy number for epidermal growth factor receptor (EGFR) and clinical response to antiEGFR treatment in colorectal cancer: a cohort study. Lancet Oncol 2005; 6: 279–86.

Pao W, Wang TY, Riely GJ, et al. *KRAS* mutations and primary resistance of lung adenocarcinomas to gefitinib or erlotinib. PLoS Med 2005; 2: e17.

Riely GJ, Pao W, Pham D, et al. Clinical course of patients with non-small cell lung cancer and epidermal growth factor receptor exon 19 and exon 21 mutations treated with gefitinib or erlotinib. Clin Cancer Res 2006; 12: 839–44.

Shepherd FA, Rodrigues PJ, Ciuleanu T, et al. Erlotinib in previously treated non-small-cell lung cancer. N Engl J Med 2005; 353: 123–32.

Safety of targeted therapies

T Macarulla, J Tabernero
Vall d'Hebron University Hospital, Barcelona, Spain

Introduction

In the last decade, the introduction of new cytotoxic agents for different tumor types has translated into a survival benefit in those patients with advanced disease and an improvement in cure rate in those treated in the adjuvant setting. The relatively non-selective cytotoxic agents have been joined recently by highly selective targeted agents. These novel drugs have improved the therapeutic index without increasing the toxic effects of cytotoxic agents, and these treatments may be better tolerated by all patients, including the elderly. Some of these agents have been approved by regulatory agencies and are used as standard treatments either as single agent or in combination with chemotherapy or radiotherapy. Nevertheless, new types of toxicity have been reported with these agents, quite different from the toxicities observed with chemotherapy.

Monoclonal antibodies

Trastuzumab

Trastuzumab was approved in 1998 as first-line treatment in combination with standard chemotherapy for HER2-positive metastatic breast cancer. The regulatory studies reported that trastuzumab was associated with two specific side-effects:

▪ hypersensibility, which was mild and mainly associated with the first infusion
▪ cardiotoxicity with congestive heart failure (CHF): cardiotoxicity has been reported in 1.4% of patients when trastuzumab is used as a single agent, but this incidence increases to 2–16% when trastuzumab is used in combination with chemotherapy, the frequency being highest among those patients receiving anthracyclines and trastuzumab simultaneously

Table 16.1 Adverse events with special focus on cardiotoxicity presented by patients with breast cancer treated in the HERA trial

Adverse event[a]	Trastuzumab[b] (N = 1677)	Observation (N = 1710)	p-value
Patients with grade 3/4 adverse events	132 (7.9%)	75 (4.4%)	<0.001
Fatal adverse event	6 (0.4%)[c]	3 (0.2%)[d]	0.34
Treatment withdrawals	143 (8.5%)[e]	—	
Cardiac events:			
Death from cardiac cause	0	1 (0.06%)	1.00
Severe CHF[f]	9 (0.54%)	0	0.002
Symptomatic CHF (including severe CHF)	29 (1.73%)	1 (0.06%)	<0.001
Decrease in LVEF[g]	113 (7.08%)	34 (2.21%)	<0.001

[a]CHF, congestive heart failure; LVEF, left ventricular ejection fraction.
[b]Limited to the group of patients treated with trastuzumab during 1 year.
[c]Cerebral hemorrhage (1 patient), cerebrovascular accident (1 patient), sudden death (1 patient), appendicitis (1 patient), and death from unknown cause (2 patients).
[d]Cardiac failure (1 patient), suicide (1 patient), unknown cause (1 patient).
[e]Adverse events (5.5%), refusal to continue (2.5%), or other (0.5%).
[f]NYHA functional class III or IV, and a decrease in the ejection fraction of 10 percentage points or more from baseline to an LVEF <50% at any time.
[g]Decrease in LVEF was defined as decrease in the ejection fraction of 10 percentage points or more from baseline to an LVEF <50% at any time.

Trastuzumab was also evaluated in an adjuvant setting in the National Surgical Adjuvant Breast and Bowel Project (NSABP) B31 Trial, the North Central Cancer Treatment Group (NCCTG) N9831 trial, and the Herceptin Adjuvant (HERA) trial.

■ The HERA trial compared either 1 or 2 years of trastuzumab with observation in patients who had completed regional treatment and adjuvant chemotherapy. In this trial, there was a low percentage of CHF compared with the data available for metastatic disease (Table 16.1). Nevertheless, these toxicity results have to be evaluated with caution due to the limited follow-up of this study.

■ In the American studies, the cumulative 3-year incidence of CHF increased by 3% with the addition of trastuzumab:
  – In the B21 study, the rate of New York Heart Association (NYHA) class III–IV CHF or death from heart disease was 0.8% in the control arm and 4.2% in the trastuzumab arm (with only one patient with persistent symptoms).
  – In the N9831 study, 0% of patients in the control arm and 2.9% (20 patients) in the trastuzumab arm had CHF (1 died of cardiomyopathy). Trastuzumab did not increase the overall frequency or severity of non-cardiac adverse events associated with chemotherapy regimens, but rare cases of interstitial pneumonitis in patients receiving trastuzumab and paclitaxel were observed, two of these cases being fatal. There is need for longer follow-up in order to define the definitive incidence of cardiac toxicity in these trials.

Cetuximab

Cetuximab is the first anti-epidermal growth factor receptor (EGFR) monoclonal antibody to be approved for cancer treatment, with a regulatory indication for irinotecan-resistant metastatic colorectal cancer (CRC).

■ In the first phase II trial, presented by Saltz et al, 121 patients with irinotecan-refractory advanced CRC were treated with cetuximab and irinotecan at the same dose and schedule that the patient had previously progressed on. The combination produced major objective responses in about 20% of patients with acceptable toxicity. Reported toxicities attributable to cetuximab were grade 3/4 allergic reactions (4%) and grade 3 rash (8%). The toxicities typically associated with irinotecan did not appear to be exacerbated by cetuximab.
■ In a second phase II study, cetuximab was used as single agent in a similar population. In this trial, 86% of patients presented skin reactions, but only 18% were grade 3. Skin reactions characteristically appeared within the first 1–3 weeks of therapy, whereas paronychial cracking, another manifestation of cetuximab-related toxicity present in 12% of patients, tended to appear later and was persistent throughout the duration of treatment. The incidence of grade 3/4 allergic reactions during infusion was 3.5%.
■ In the BOND study, 329 irinotecan-resistant CRC patients were randomized to receive cetuximab plus irinotecan or single-agent cetuximab. Cetuximab showed antitumor activity both as a single agent and in combination with irinotecan. In this study, 80% of patients in each group developed an

Adverse event, grade 3/4	Cetuximab plus irinotecan (N = 212)	Cetuximab, single agent (N = 115)	p-value
Any	138 (65.1%)	50 (43.5%)	<0.001
Anemia	10 (4.7%)	3 (2.6%)	0.55
Neutropenia	20 (9.4%)	0	<0.001
Thrombocytopenia	1 (0.5%)	1 (0.9%)	1.00
Diarrhea	45 (21.2%)	2 (1.7%)	<0.001
Asthenia	29 (13.7%)	12 (10.4%)	0.49
Acne-like rash	20 (9.4%)	6 (5.2%)	0.20
Nausea and vomiting	15 (7.1%)	5 (4.3%)	0.47
Abdominal pain	7 (3.3%)	6 (5.2%)	0.39
Stomatitis	5 (2.4%)	1 (0.9%)	0.67
Dyspnea	3 (1.4%)	15 (13.0%)	<0.001
Fever	5 (2.4%)	0	0.17
Hypersensitivity reaction	0	4 (3.5%)	0.01
Death	0	0	1.00

acne-like rash, but only 9.4% in the combination group and 5.2% in the single-agent arm presented grade 3 rash; 1.2% of patients developed a severe anaphylactic reaction to cetuximab. The rates of incidence of other hematological and non-hematological toxic effects in the combination group were similar to those reported in studies with irinotecan as a second-line treatment (Table 16.2).

In all three studies, there was a correlation between the presence of skin rash and overall survival. Patients with a skin rash had a superior survival compared with those patients without rash.

Another adverse event that may be present in patients treated with cetuximab is hypomagnesemia, the mechanism of which is not clear. Some patients, depending on the severity, can present clinical symptoms.

Table 16.3 Adverse events presented in metastatic colorectal cancer patients treated with IFL[a] with or without bevacizumab as first-line treatment

Adverse event	IFL[a] plus placebo (N = 397)	IFL plus bevacizumab (N = 393)
Any grade 3/4 adverse event	74.0%	84.9%
Grade 3/4 leukopenia	31.1%	37.0%
Grade 3/4 diarrhea	24.7%	32.4%
Grade 3 hypertension	2.3%	11.0%
Any thrombotic event	16.2%	19.4%
Deep thrombophlebitis	6.3%	8.9%
Pulmonary embolus	5.1%	3.6%
Grade 3/4 bleeding	2.5%	3.1%
Grade 3 proteinuria	0.8%	0.8%
Gastrointestinal perforation	0.0%	1.5%

[a]Irinotecan, 5-fluorouracil, leucovorin (folinic acid).

Bevacizumab

Colorectal cancer

Bevacizumab, a monoclonal antibody directed against the vascular endothelial growth factor (VEGF), was approved by the European Medicines Agency (EMEA) in 2005 as first-line treatment of advanced CRC in combination with irinotecan- and 5-fluorouracil (5-FU)-based chemotherapy.

■ Hurwitz et al reported the results of the first phase III study using bevacizumab in combination with chemotherapy in previously untreated metastatic CRC. These patients were randomized to receive either irinotecan, 5-FU, and leucovorin (folinic acid) (IFL) plus bevacizumab (5 mg/kg) or IFL alone. The combination treatment resulted in statistically significant improvements in response rate, time to progression, and overall survival. Previous phase I and II trials had reported rare but serious bevacizumab-related toxicities: hemorrhage, thromboembolism, gastrointestinal perforation, proteinuria, and hypertension. In this phase III study, these side-effects were observed, but only the incidence of grade 3 hypertension was clearly significantly increased in the bevacizumab arm (Table 16.3).

Table 16.4 Safety results of the E3200 study in patients with advanced colorectal cancer treated in the second-line setting with FOLFOX 4[a] plus bevacizumab, FOLFOX 4 without bevacizumab, or bevacizumab monotherapy

Adverse event, grade 3/4 toxicity	FOLFOX[a] 4 plus bevacizumab (N=287)	FOLFOX 4 (N=287)	Bevacizumab (N=234)
Hypertension	6%	3%	7%
Bleeding	3%	<1%	2%
Neuropathy	16%	9%	2%
Vomiting	10%	4%	5%
Proteinuria	1%	0%	<1%
Hematemesis	2%	0%	2%
Melena/gastrointestinal bleeding	6%	1%	1%
Venous thrombosis	10%	7%	1%
Cardiac ischemia	3%	1%	1%
Cerebrovascular ischemia	1%	0%	0%
Bowel perforation	1%	0%	1.3%

[a]Oxaliplatin, 5-fluorouracil, leucovorin (folinic acid).

■ Giantonio et al randomized patients with previously treated metastatic CRC to FOLFOX 4 (oxaliplatin, 5-FU, and leucovorin), FOLFOX 4 plus bevacizumab (10 mg/kg), or bevacizumab alone. Bevacizumab plus FOLFOX 4 improved overall survival, time to progression, and response rate. The treatment was well tolerated; hypertension and bleeding were more common in the combination arm. Bowel perforation, although infrequent, was only present in the bevacizumab arms (Table 16.4).

■ The TREE 1 and 2 studies assessed the safety and efficacy of bevacizumab when added to an oxaliplatin/fluoropyrimidine regimen as first-line treatment in metastatic CRC. The addition of bevacizumab to chemotherapy increased the rate of grade 3/4 hypertension and impaired wound healing, and was associated with bowel perforation (Table 16.5). The authors concluded that the grade 3/4 toxicities present in the patients treated with first-line bevacizumab plus oxaliplatin-based therapy was acceptable.

■ BRITE and BEAT are two observational studies of bevacizumab with different chemotherapy schedules in first-line treatment of patients with advanced CRC. The objective of these two studies was to evaluate the safety profile of bevacizumab with these schedules. In the BRITE study, 1968 patients were followed for up to 3 years. Bevacizumab-related serious adverse events were reported in 12% of patients, the most relevant being:
  – gastrointestinal perforation (1.7%)
  – postoperative bleeding or wound healing complications (1.2%)
  – arterial thromboembolic events (2.1%)
  – grade 3/4 bleeding (1.9%)

In the BEAT study, after a follow-up of 13 months, the most common grade 3–4 side effects related to bevacizumab were: bleeding (2.1%), gastrointestinal perforation (1.6%), arterial thromboembolic events (0.9%), wound healing complications, and hypertension (3.7%).

Non-small cell lung cancer

The addition of bevacizumab to standard first-line chemotherapy in patients with advanced non-squamous non-small cell lung cancer (NSCLC) has translated into improved survival.

■ The first randomized phase II study, by Johnson et al, compared bevacizumab (at either 7.5 mg/kg or 15 mg/kg) plus carboplatin and paclitaxel with the same chemotherapy schedule in previously untreated locally advanced or metastatic NSCLC. The group treated with bevacizumab at 15 mg/kg showed improvements in response rate, time to progression, and survival compared with the control arm. The addition of bevacizumab to chemotherapy resulted in only modest changes in the expected toxicity profile with chemotherapy alone. Slightly higher toxicity was observed in terms of leukopenia, diarrhea, and minor systemic events (fever, headache, rash, and chills). Certain bevacizumab-associated adverse events were of particular significance, namely hypertension, proteinuria, and bleeding.
  – Grade 3 hypertension (defined as requiring new or increased antihypertensive medical therapy) was observed in the high-dose arm (2 patients); however, no patients in this trial discontinued bevacizumab because of hypertension.
  – Asymptomatic proteinuria (determined by dipstick analysis) was observed in 21 patients in the bevacizumab arms (7 in the low-dose arm, 14 in the high-dose arm) and 2 in the control arm.
  – Two clinically distinct patterns of bleeding were observed during the study: minor mucosal hemorrhage and major hemoptysis. The most

Adverse event, grade 3/4	mFOLFOX-bev[a] (N=71)	bFOL-bev[b] (N=70)	CapeOx-bev[c] (N=72)
Any	85%	74%	76%
Nausea	6%	11%	11%
Vomiting	1%	13%	10%
Dehydration	6%	14%	8%
Diarrhea	13%	26%	19%
Hypertension	7%	13%	15%
Arterial thromboembolic events	0%	0%	3%
Other thromboembolic events	10%	10%	4%
Neurotoxicity	14%	11%	15%
Hand-foot	0%	0%	10%
Neutropenia	49%	19%	10%
Sepsis (all grades)	4.2%	4.3%	1.4%
Bowel perforation (all grades)	4.2%	2.9%	2.8
Impaired wound healing (all grades)	5.6%	1.4%	5.6%
Treatment-related deaths	0%	4.3%	4.2%

mFOLFOX: oxaliplatin 85 mg/m^2, leucovorin (folinic acid, LV) 350 mg/m^2, 5-fluorouracil (5-FU) bolus 400 mg/m^2 and 2400 mg/m^2 continuous intravently infusion during 48 h q2wk.
bFOL: oxaliplatin 85 mg/m^2 d1 and 15, LV 20 mg/m^2 and bolus 5-FU 500 mg/m^2 d1, 8, 15 q4wk.
CapeOx: oxaliplatin 130 mg/m^2 d1, capecitabine 1000 mg/m^2 bid (850 mg/m^2 for TREE 2) for 14 days q3wk.
bev: bevacizumab added to each regimen (5 mg/kg q2wk or 7.5 mg/kg q3wk).

common mucocutaneous bleeding was grade 1/2 epistaxis (31% in the low-dose arm and 44% in the high-dose arm, compared with 6% in the control arm); none required modifications in bevacizumab administration. Six patients experienced a major life-threatening bleeding, described as hemoptysis or hematemesis, and 4 of these cases were fatal. All 6 patients had centrally located tumors close to major vessels, 5 had cavitations or necrosis in the tumor, and 4 had squamous cell histology. The authors concluded that as squamous cell tumors are more frequently centrally located and have a greater tendency to cavitate as compared with adenocarcinomas, it is not clear whether histology alone is the central risk factor for bleeding or simply a surrogate for other risk factors.

■ In a phase III study published by Sandler et al, 878 patients with advanced non-squamous NSCLC were randomized to receive paclitaxel plus carboplatin with or without bevacizumab at 15 mg/kg. The addition of bevacizumab to standard chemotherapy in this group of patients provided a statistically and clinically significant survival advantage, with manageable toxicity (Table 16.6). The authors concluded that bevacizumab used in a low-risk bleeding population was associated with a limited increase in serious bleeding, including hemoptysis.

Summary

Monoclonal antibodies thus have a class-related toxicity (hypersensitivity reactions) and a target-related toxicity. The latter is dependent on the target:

■ HER2/*neu*: cardiotoxicity
■ EGFR: skin toxicity
■ VEGF: hypertension, proteinuria, thromboembolism, and bleeding complications

Small molecules

Erlotinib

The US Food and Drug Administration (FDA) and the EMEA have approved erlotinib for the treatment of patients with NSCLC as a second- or third-line therapy. This approval was the result of the National Cancer Institute of Canada (NCIC) phase III trial published by Shepherd et al in patients with stage IIIB or IV NSCLC who had progressed to one or two prior regimens of chemotherapy and were randomized to receive placebo or erlotinib. Erlotinib significantly prolonged survival compared with the placebo arm. The toxic effects were mild, with 5% of patients discontinuing the treatment due to drug-related toxic effects. The most frequent grade 3/4 adverse events in the erlotinib arm were rash (9%) and diarrhea (6%), with 19% of patients in the erlotinib group requiring dose reduction, mostly due to rash and

Table 16.6 Safety results of the E4599 study in patients with advanced non-small cell lung cancer: patients were randomized to receive carboplatin and paclitaxel with or without bevacizumab

Adverse event, grade ≥ 3	Paclitaxel/ carboplatin (N = 440)	Paclitaxel/ carboplatin plus bevacizumab (N = 420)	P value[a]
Neutropenia	16.8%	25.5%	0.002
Thrombocytopenia	0.2%	1.6%	0.04
Anemia	0.9%	0%	NS
Febrile neutropenia	1.8%	4%	0.02
Hypertension	0.7%	7%	<0.001
Proteinuria	0%	3.1%	<0.001
Bleeding events (all)	0.7%	4.4%	<0.01
Central nervous system	0%	0.7%	
Epistaxis	0.2%	0.7%	
Hematemesis	0%	0.5%	
Hemptysis	0.2%	1.9%	
Gastrointestinal bleeding	0.4%	0.9%	
Other hemorrhage	0%	0.4%	

[a]NS, not statistically significant.

diarrhea. There were similar rates of pneumonitis and pulmonary fibrosis in the two groups (<1%). Erlotinib was not associated with notable myelotoxicity, even in patients with extensive prior chemotherapy. Hepatic abnormalities were mild (grade 1 or 2), even in patients with elevated liver function tests at baseline.

In summary, rash and diarrhea are characteristic side-effects of erlotinib. Life-threatening toxicities, such as interstitial pneumonia, were rarely observed with erlotinib.

The FDA and EMEA have approved the combination of erlotinib with gemcitabine in patients with metastatic pancreatic cancer based on the results of a phase III study in 569 patients with advanced untreated pancreatic cancer.

Patients were randomized to receive gemcitabine plus erlotinib or gemcitabine alone. The combination of gemcitabine plus erlotinib slightly but significantly improved survival and progression-free survival as compared with gemcitabine alone.

There was an increased incidence of grade 3/4 rash (6% vs 1%) and diarrhea (6% vs 2%) in the erlotinib arm. Other rates of grade 3/4 toxicities were comparable in both arms.

In this study, patients with grade ≥ 2 rash presented a statistically significant better median survival and 1-year survival compared with patients with grade < 2 rash. The increased toxicity associated with erlotinib was considered as tolerable, and the presence of grade ≥ 2 rash was a predictive factor of response.

Gefitinib

Gefitinib has been approved in Japan and the US as second-line treatment in patients with NSCLC. A phase III trial by Thatcher et al in patients with refractory advanced NSCLC treated with gefitinib or best supportive care only did not show any advantage in survival in the gefitinib arm. Adverse events were more frequently observed in the gefitinib group, consisting of grade 3/4 rash (3%) and grade 3/4 diarrhea (2%). In this study, the incidence of interstitial lung disease was similar in the two treatment groups (1%), patients of Asiatic origin having a higher incidence than the rest of the population.

Imatinib

Imatinib mesylate is approved worldwide for use in gastrointestinal stromal tumors (GIST), with a recommended dose of 400 mg daily. It is a protein tyrosine kinase inhibitor that inhibits Abl, c-Kit and the platelet-derived growth factor receptor (PDGFR). This drug was highly active in patients with c-KIT-positive GIST in phase II studies. The treatment was well tolerated at a dose of 400 mg daily. The most frequent side-effects were anemia (92%), edema (particularly periorbital edema) (84%), skin rash (69%), fatigue (76%), nausea (57%), granulocytopenia (43%), and diarrhea (47%). Most of these side-effects were mild to moderate and tended to occur in the first 8 weeks of treatment.

In two randomized trials, two doses of imatinib were compared (400 mg daily and 800 mg daily) for the treatment of advanced GIST. The toxicity rates reported in these trials were similar to those in the previous phase II studies (Table 16.7).

Adverse event, grade 1–4	Imatinib 400 mg	Imatinib 800 mg
Anemia	89.9%	97.2%
Granulcytopenia	43.1%	44.3%
Edema	73.1%	87.3%
Skin rash	29.3%	45.5%
Fatigue	69.2%	77.5%
Nausea	51.5%	59.2%
Vomiting	28.4%	36.3%
Diarrhea	49.4%	55.2%
Bleeding	12.6%	20.4%

Multityrosine kinase inhibitors

Sorafenib

Sorafenib is a tyrosine kinase inhibitor active against Raf, the VEGF receptor (VEGFR), PDGFR, Flt3, and c-Kit. This drug has demonstrated antitumoral activity in renal cell carcinoma (RCC). In a randomized phase III study, 769 patients who had received one prior systemic therapy for advanced RCC were randomized to received sorafenib or best supportive care. Any grade 3/4 events were reported in 30% of patients in the sorafenib arm and in 22% in the placebo arm. The most relevant adverse events in the sorafenib arm were hypertension (1%), fatigue (2%), diarrhea (1%), rash (1%), and hand–foot syndrome (5%). Sorafinib significantly prolonged progression-free survival compared to placebo.

Sunitinib

Sunitinib is another multitargeted tyrosine kinase inhibitor. This drug has its antitumor activity through inhibition of PDGFR, VEGFR, c-Kit and Flt3. Two sequentially conducted single-arm, multicenter phase II trials have confirmed antitumor activity of sunitinib in patients with metastatic RCC as second-line therapy. The most relevant grade 3 adverse events reported in these trials were neutropenia (13%), thrombocytopenia (6% in trial 2), fatigue (11% in trial 1 and 8% in trial 2), diarrhea (3% in both trials), stomatitis (2% in trial 1 and 5% in trial 2), left ventricular ejection fraction (LVEF) decline (2% in both trials), and hypertension (2–6%).

Motzer et al presented in the 2006 ASCO meeting the results of a phase III trial that has permitted the approval of sunitinib in the US and Europe for the first-line treatment of metastatic RCC. A total of 750 untreated metastatic RCC patients were randomized to received sunitinib or interferon-alfa. This trial demonstrated a statistically significant improvement in progression-free survival and objective response rate for the sunitinib arm over the interferon-alfa arm. The treatment with sunitinib was well tolerated (Table 16.8).

Table 16.8 Treatment-related adverse events in the phase III trial of sunitinib in patients with first-line treatment metastatic RCC presented in the 2006 ASCO meeting

Adverse event, grade ≥3	Sunitinib (N=375)	IFN-α (N=375)
Neutropenia	12%	7%
Anemia	3%	4%
Thrombocytopenia	8%	0%
Lymphopenia	12%	22%
Fatigue	7%	11%
Diarrhea	5%	0%
Nausea	3%	1%
Stomatitis	1%	<1%
Hypertension	8%	<1%
Ejection fraction decline	2%	1%
Pyrexia	1%	0%
Chills	1%	0%
Myalgia	<1%	<1%
Flu-like symptoms	0%	<1%

IFN-α: Interferon-alfa

Conclusions

Targeted agents are currently emerging as new cancer treatments, with several currently approved specific indications. Novel targeted agents aim to interfere with specific critical properties of malignant cells, with limited impact on the non-neoplastic host cells, thereby increasing the therapeutic index in comparison with conventional cytotoxic agents. However, most targeted agents have the best therapeutic effect when they are used in combination with standard chemotherapy. Therefore, the specific toxicities related to targeted agents have to be analyzed in combination with the toxicities related to cytotoxic agents.

Although molecular targeted agents differ in their mechanism of action, they do not have a unique toxicity profile:

- ■ EGFR-targeting agents are associated with skin and nail toxicity, and less frequently with diarrhea.
- ■ Agents directed to inhibit angiogenesis are commonly associated with hypertension and proteinuria, and less frequently with hemorrhage, thrombotic arterial events, and gastrointestinal perforation.

The information emerging from prospective randomized studies is increasingly establishing the toxicity profile related to the administration of these targeted agents.

Further reading

Cunningham D, Humblet Y, Siena S, et al. Cetuximab monotherapy and cetuximab plus irinotecan in irinotecan-refractory metastatic colorectal cancer. N Engl J Med 2004; 351: 337–45.

Escudier B, Szczylik C, Eisen T, et al. Randomized phase III of the Raf kinase and VEGFR inhibitor sorafenib (BAY-43-9006) in patients with advanced renal cell carcinoma. Proc Am Soc Clin Oncol 2005; 22: 4510a.

Hochster HS, Hart LL, Ramanathan RK, et al. Safety and efficacy of oxaliplatin-fluoropyrimidine regimens with or without bevacizumaa as first-line treatment of metastatic colorectal cancer (MCRC): Final analysis of the TREE study. Proc Am Soc Clin Oncol 2006; 148s: 310a.

Hurwitz H, Fehrenbacher L, Novotny W, et al. Bevacizumab plus irinotecan, fluorouracil, and leucovorin for metastatic colorectal cancer. N Engl J Med 2004; 350: 2335–42.

Johnson DH, Fehrenbacher L, Novotny WF, et al. Randomized phase II trial comparing bevacizumab plus carboplatin and paclitaxel with carboplatin and paclitaxel alone in previously untreated locally advanced or metastatic non-small-cell lung cancer. J Clin Oncol 2004; 22: 2184–91.

Kozloff M, Hainsworth J, Badrinath S, et al. Safety and efficacy of bevacizumab plus chemotherapy as first-line treatment of patients with metastatic colorectal cancer: Updated results from a large observational registry in the US (Brite). Proc ESMO 2006 meeting; abstract 0–018.

Moore MJ, Goldstein D, Hamm J, et al. Erlotinib plus gemcitabine compared to gemcitabine alone in patients with advanced pancreatic cancer. A phase III trial of the

National Cancer Institute of Canada Clinical Trials Group. Proc Am Soc Clin Oncol 2005; 25: 1a.

Motzer RJ, Hutson TE, Tomczak P, et al. Phase III randomized trial of sunitinib malate (SU11248) versus interferon-alfa as first-line systemic therapy for patients with metastatic renal cell carcinoma. Proc Am Soc Clin Oncol 2006; 2s: 3a.

Piccart-Gebhart MJ, Procter M, Leyland-Jones B, et al. Trastuzumab after adjuvant chemotherapy in HER2-positive breast cancer. N Engl J Med 2005; 353: 1659–72.

Romond EH, Perez EA, Bryant J, et al. Trastuzumab plus adjuvant chemotherapy for operable HER2-positive breast cancer. N Engl J Med 2005; 353: 1673–84.

Saltz L, Meropol NJ, Loehrer PJ, et al. Phase II trial of cetuximab in patients with refractory colorectal cancer that expresses the epidermal growth factor receptor. J Clin Oncol 2004; 22: 1201–8.

Sandler A, Gray R, Perry MC, et al. Paclitaxel-Carboplatin alone or with bevacizumab for non-small-cell lung cancer. N Engl J Med 2006; 355: 2542–50.

Saltz L, Rubin M, Hochster H, et al. Cetuximab plus irinotecan is active in CPT-11-refractory colorectal cancer that expresses Epidermal Growth Factor Receptor. Proc Am Soc Clin Oncol 2001; 22: 7a.

Schrag D, Chung KY, Flombaum C, Saltz L. Cetuximab therapy and symptomatic hypomagnesemia. J Natl Cancer Inst 2005; 97: 1221-4.

Shepherd FA, Rodrigues Pereira J, Ciuleanu T, et al. Erlotinib in previously treated non-small cell lung cancer. N Engl J Med 2005; 353: 123–32.

Slamon D, Leyland-Jones B, Shak S, et al. Use of chemotherapy plus a monoclonal antibody against HER2 for metastatic breast cancer that overexpresses HER2. N Engl J Med 2001; 344: 783–92.

Thatcher N, Chang A, Parikh P, et al. Gefitinib plus best supportive care in previously treated patients with refractory advanced non-small-cell lung cancer: results from a randomized, placebo-controlled, multicentre study (Iressa Survival Evaluation in Lung Cancer). Lancet 2005; 366: 1527–37.

Townsley CA, Pond GR, Oza AM, et al. Evaluation of adverse events experienced by older patients participating in studies of molecularly targeted agents alone or in combination. Clin Cancer Res 2006; 12: 2141–9.

Van Cutsem E, Michael M, Berry S, et al. Preliminary safety and efficacy of beva-cizumab with first-line FOLFOX, XELOX, FOLFIRI, and capecitabine for mCRC: first BEAT trial. Proc Gastrointestinal Am Soc Clin Oncol meeting 2007; 23: 3460.

Verweij J, Oosterom A, Blay J, et al. Imatinib mesylate is an active agent for gastrointestinal stroma tumors, but does not yield responses in other soft-tissue sarcomas that are unselected for molecular target: results from an EORTC Soft Tissue and Bone Sarcoma Group phase II study. Eur J Cancer 2003; 39: 2006-11.

Functional immunology and biomarkers

M Palma, H Mellstedt, A Choudhury
Karolinska University Hospital, Stockholm, Sweden

17

Introduction

Biomarkers are biomolecules such as messenger ribonucleic acid (mRNA), proteins, or peptides that can be quantitated to evaluate different disease-related variables, including the outcome of a treatment.

Biomarkers available in tumor immunology measure various components of the immune system. They are usually employed either to identify novel tumor-associated antigens (TAAs) with immunogenic properties to be targeted in a vaccination approach or as surrogate endpoints to evaluate the efficacy of a vaccine.

For the latter purpose, both B-cell and T-cell biomarkers are used for the assessment of vaccine-induced humoral and cellular immunity, respectively. A pre-vaccine versus post-vaccine comparison of antitumor immune response gives information on the immunological efficacy of the vaccine (vaccine potency).

As for every anticancer treatment, the primary endpoints of a vaccine treatment are survival and time-to-disease progression, tumor regression and improvement of quality of life.

The induction of a specific, long-lasting immune response can be regarded as a surrogate endpoint for clinical outcome after vaccination. However, as with other such surrogate endpoints (e.g., elimination of micrometastasis and changes in tumor markers), the clinical relevance of a vaccine-induced immune response has not yet been established.

Fundamental considerations for measuring antitumor responses

Generally, the antitumor immune response should be T helper 1 (T_{h1}) type, involving both humoral and cellular arms and activating the innate as well as adaptive immune system.

Unlike vaccines against infectious diseases, which are primarily measured with humoral markers, the success of an anticancer vaccination approach is essentially assessed by cellular immunological biomarkers. This is because a T-cell-mediated immune response is thought to be the most effective to eradicate tumors in vivo.

Unlike antibody responses, however, which can be easily detected and titrated in peripheral blood, antigen (Ag)-specific lymphocytes may not be easily detectable in peripheral blood. Although it has been proven that Ag-specific lymphocytes can also be found in tumor tissue, bone marrow, and regional lymph nodes, peripheral blood is the only compartment accessible for serial analyses in a clinical setting. The only in vivo measure of Ag-specific immunity is the delayed-type hypersensitivity (DTH) test. All other measurements are performed in vitro.

■ The first generation of ex vivo T-cell assays includes lymphoproliferation assays and cytotoxicity assays against tumor targets using a radioactive isotope of chromium (^{51}Cr). Like DTH, these assays measure overall T-cell response before and after vaccination.

■ Second-generation T-cell assays, on the other hand, measure the immune response at the individual immune cell level. Detecting single-cell events, they produce quantitative and qualitative data; i.e., they provide individual cell phenotypic and functional information. They include both peptide major histocompatibility complex (MHC) tetramers and detection of cytokines by different assays, the most common of which are enzyme-linked immunospot (ELISPOT), cytokine flow cytometry (CFC), and real-time polymerase chain reaction (PCR). In general, these assays are very sensitive to variations in assay conditions, and their sensitivity can be impaired by non-specific background cytokine production, but ELISPOT and CFC have now used extensively, and provide information that can be quite reliably correlated with treatment clinical efficacy.

■ Third-generation assays represent an evolution of the second-generation ones. After detecting specific T cells with tetramers or CFC, they characterize T-cell properties such as cytotoxic, proliferative, and migratory capacity, regulatory functions, and the ability of T cells to interact with other cells of the immune system, such as antigen-presenting cells (APC). These assays allow functional evaluation of different T-cell subpopulations (e.g., memory, helper, and cytotoxic T cells), either at the T-cell receptor (TCR) level (TCR affinity or avidity) or by measuring their cytokine production in response to Ag exposure. Nevertheless, as no specific correlation has yet been found between any of these T-cell properties and clinical vaccine efficacy, third-generation assays need further validation.

Advantages and disadvantages of these assays are shown in Table 17.1.

Clinical implications

Some immunological parameters have been shown to correlate with improved prognosis, including: MHC class II expression on tumor cells; extensive intratumoral infiltration of CD8+ T cells, dendritic cells (DC), natural killer (NK) cells, macrophages, and eosinophils; and the presence of CD8+ tumor-infiltrating lymphocytes (TIL) showing proliferative activity and interferon-γ (IFN-γ) secretion.

In contrast, there have also been indications in certain malignancies that an abundant infiltration of tumor tissue by CD8+ and CD4+ T cells is associated with shorter survival, while a high frequency of CD8+ Ki-67+ TIL (proliferating cells) is associated with longer survival. Nevertheless, the use of these parameters as clinical correlates has to be regarded as premature.

Clinical use

At present, no single validated and quality-assured method has been proven to be an accurate and reproducible indicator of clinical prognosis following anticancer vaccination therapy. The accuracy and reproducibility of all available T-cell-based methods is still suboptimal, and assays combining enumeration of activated T cells with functional antitumor activity have to be further validated.

Serological tests are undoubtedly less problematic, and analysis of immunoglobulin G (IgG) subclass response might be useful, but, for the reasons mentioned above, they are less informative than cellular tests with regard to antitumor immune response.

At present, for immune monitoring of vaccine clinical trials, it is recommended that a combination of two or more second-generation assays should be used and that their cumulative findings could be utilized as indicators of immunological activation following vaccine therapy.

The field of biomarkers for immunological monitoring is still nascent and rapidly developing. The key issues are: the delineation of in vitro assays that demonstrate accurate and reproducible correlation with clinical prognosis,

Table 17.1 T-cell assays used for immune monitoring

Assay	Brief description	Advantages	Disadvantages
Delayed-type hypersensitivity (DTH)	Ag as soluble protein is injected intradermally and the diameter of erythema or induration is measured after 48–72 h	• The only in vivo measure available • Easy to perform	• No standardized cut-off for a positive response • No standardized dose for DTH testing • Ag-specificity is questionable
Lymphoproliferation assay	Lymphocytes are cultured with the Ag studied. [³H]thymidine is added to the culture medium. Proliferating (dividing) cells which incorporate [³H]thymidine, which is quantitated using a β scintillation counter	• Easy to perform • Reliable • Sensitive • Reproducible	• Can be influenced by the non-specific immune function of the patient • Can be influenced by the in vitro stimulation procedure • Not qualitative • Not quantitative • No information about responding cell population (CD4⁺, CD8⁺, etc.)

(Continued)

Table 17.1 Continued

Assay	Brief description	Advantages	Disadvantages
Cytotoxicity assay	Lymphocytes previously sensitized to the Ag present on the target cells are co-cultured with the target cells. Percentage of lysis of target cells is quantitated by ^{57}Cr release assay or flow cytometry	• Functional assay • Measures the capability of direct tumor lysis	• Low sensitivity • Often involves multiple in vitro stimulations • Not quantitative • Often other targets than autologous tumor are used, which may not reflect the capability of effector cells to lyse autologous tumor cells in vivo
Enzyme-linked immunospot (ELISPOT)	Lymphocytes are cultured with the Ag and studied in a microtiter plate coated with a monoclonal Ab to a specific soluble factor (e.g. IFN-γ, IL-4, IL-10, TNF-α). The cells and	• Functional assay • Allows measurement of individual soluble factors secreted by activated T cells and identification of the pathway	• Provides no information on cell phenotype

Table 17.1 Continued

Assay	Brief description	Advantages	Disadvantages
	the Ag are then washed from the wells and replaced with a secondary Ab conjugated to a detection reagent. The plate is developed with a chromogen, and spots appear where there was a cell secreting the soluble factor being investigated	of the immune system activated by the vaccine • Lowest limit of detection ($1/10^5$ Ag-specific T cells) • Considerably reliable • Relatively rapid	
Tetramer staining	Tetramers are composed of four MHC-I molecules, each bound to the epitope of interest. The tag is a fluorescent label, which allows measurement of the binding of the tetramer to the TCR on flow cytometry	• Sensitive ($1/10^4$ Ag-specific T cells) • T-cell subset analysis is optimal • Allows identification of the peptide sequence or epitopes that bind to the highest number of TCRs in a naive individual	• Requires knowledge of the epitope • Requires availability of the tetramer for the respective epitope/HLA allele • Unable to distinguish between functional and dysfunctional T cells

(Continued)

Table 17.1 Continued

Assay	Brief description	Advantages	Disadvantages
		• Allows identification of the phenotype of the T cell to which the tetramer binds	
		• Allows measurement of the change in the number of T cells displaying a particular TCR before and after vaccination	
Cytokine flow cytometry	Lymphocytes are cultured with the Ag studied, and the presence of intracellular cytokines is detected by a fluorescein-labeled mAb. The phenotype of the lymphoid cells (CD4$^+$, CD8$^+$,	• Functional assay • Sensitive (1/10^4 Ag-specific T cells) • Provides additional information on cell phenotypes	• Non-specific background staining

(Continued)

163

Table 17.1 Continued

Assay	Brief description	Advantages	Disadvantages
	etc.) is identified with a second set of fluorescein-labeled mAbs	• Relatively rapid	
Real-time polymerase chain reaction (PCR)	Detection and quantitation of cytokines at the DNA/RNA level	• Very sensitive (1/20 000– 1/50 000 Ag-specific T cells) • Quantitative • Flexible • Least specimen required • Does not require in vitro expansion	• Lack of standardization • Does not measure cytokines at protein level • Cannot quantitate T-cell frequencies or characterize T cells • Time-consuming

Ag, antigen; Ab, antibody; IFN-γ, interferon-γ; IL, interleukin; TNF-α, tumor necrosis factor α; MHC-I, major histocompatibility complex class I; TCR, T-cell receptor; mAb: monoclonal antibody.

standardization of the assay protocols to eliminate inter-laboratory variability, and resolution of issues with regard to the sampling of circulating peripheral blood cells, although the immune effectors may reside in other components. It is anticipated that large-scale studies and new and improved approaches for sampling immune cells and assaying immune biomarkers may lead to the development of a set of standard criteria for measuring immunological function after anticancer vaccination.

Further reading

Hogrefe WR. Biomarkers and assessment of vaccine responses. Biomarkers 2005; 10(Suppl 1): S50–7.

Keilholz U, Martus P, Scheibenbogen C. Immune monitoring of T-cell responses in cancer vaccine development. Clin Cancer Res 2006; 12: 2346s–52s.

Knutson KL, de la Rosa C, Disis ML. Laboratory analysis of T-cell immunity. Front Biosci 2006; 11: 1932–44.

Assessment of protein profiles (proteomics) as biomarkers

18

H Zwierna, J Loeffler-Ragg

Introduction

The development of the anticancer drugs is currently undergoing fundamental changes. Due to the increasing understanding of the mechanisms relevant to the genesis of cancer, there is a transition from disease-oriented to target-oriented therapy. Thus, the challenge of bringing new therapeutics to clinical application and registration now focuses on the molecular target expressed by the malignant cell rather than on treatment of the histopathological entity itself.

The new concepts, however, bring major problems for clinical drug development. One major issue is, on the one hand, the limited availability of predictive in vitro models and, on the other, the need to perform early clinical trials, usually in heavily pretreated patients with a considerable tumor load. Maximum tolerated dose (MTD) and response rate, however, are no longer the only decision-making endpoints of phase I/II trials. The new generation of compounds usually exhibit only limited toxicity and, in the vast majority of patients, stabilize the tumor rather than leading to massive reduction of tumor load. Therefore, additional endpoints different from those used for cytotoxic drugs need to be established in order to define subgroups of patients who will or will not profit from therapy.

Use of biomarkers in drug development

Biomarkers serve as hallmarks for the status of tumor growth at a given time, and change during the disease process. Their use for the detection of progressive disease or the definition of subpopulations of patients is not new:

- Increase in prostate-specific antigen (PSA) during or after therapy points to disease progression in prostate cancer.
- Evaluation of estrogen and progesterone receptors is crucial to define the optimum treatment of breast cancer.

The first drug to be registered that was based on target expression was trastuzumab (Herceptin). It is important to note that the development of trastuzumab would have failed if it had been developed without knowledge of patients' HER2 status. Another more recent example is the development of tyrosine kinase (TK) inhibitors directed against the epidermal growth factor receptor (EGFR). Activating mutations in the TK domain of the receptor leads to enhanced TK activity in response to ligand binding, and can predict response to therapy with TK inhibitors.

- Biomarkers can be used to define subgroups of patients whose tumors express a specific target and thus may have a high probability of response.
- They provide a chance to allow proof of principle in early clinical trials in order to move rapidly to phase III trials and registration.
- They can help to understand the mechanism of action of an agent. This is crucial, because more and more molecularly targeted drugs enter combination trials before in-depth knowledge of their efficacy and mode of action as single agents has been obtained and before potential resistance mechanisms have been investigated.

Despite the enormous progress in molecularly targeted therapy, in some cases clinical development of active agents may have failed in the past and may fail in the future due to lack of availability of biomarkers:

- The matrix metalloproteinase inhibitors (MMPs) showed no benefit in phase III trials despite very encouraging results from early clinical trials. It is probable that these agents have only been negative in phase III because of heterogeneous target expression similar to what would have happened had the pivotal trastuzumab trials also included HER2-negative patients.

With the rapidly growing understanding of the molecular biology of cancer, it is thus crucial to define, evaluate, and validate additional biomarkers that at a later stage of clinical development may become surrogate markers and thus add to conventional endpoints such as tumor shrinkage or disease progression (Table 18.1).

Despite much progress, biomarker development is still at an early stage, and, whenever possible, material from study patients must be stored to allow its evaluation at a later stage.

Table 18.1 Definition of endpoints in clinical trials

Clinical endpoint
Characteristic or variable, reflecting how a patient feels or functions or how long a patient survives
Biomarker
Indicator of normal biological/pathogenic processes or a pharmacological response to a therapeutic intervention
Surrogate marker
Biomarker intended to substitute for/add to a clinical endpoint

Functional imaging for the development of anti-angiogenic agents

One of the key questions relating to the development of anti-angiogenic agents is how to identify their optimum dose and schedule as single drugs and then proceed to combination schedules. Therefore, a large amount of work has been devoted to identifying and validating biological pharmacodynamic endpoints that could be used to optimize the development of anti-angiogenic drugs. While measurement of serum levels of cytokines involved in angiogenesis has been shown to be of minor relevance, potential effects of anti-angiogenic compounds can be monitored by functional imaging, and various methods have been evaluated:

■ The most widespread method is dynamic contrast-enhanced magnetic resonance imaging (DCE-MRI), since vascular permeability is a surrogate for angiogenesis and can be assessed by MRI scanning. With this imaging technique, a marked heterogeneity in drug distribution and clearance has been shown among different patients and even when deposits of tumor have been compared in the same patient. Given these significant biological differences in intratumoral drug pharmacokinetics and biological response, a major effort and emphasis needs to be put on the investigation of functional imaging as a pharmacodynamic biomarker.

This is of major clinical relevance, as effective treatment in some patients requires higher doses than in others since the optimal biologically active dose varies among individual patients.

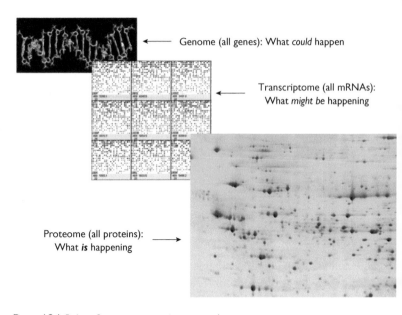

Figure 18.1 Roles of genome, transcriptome, and proteome

Assessment of proteins

Given the shortcomings of single tumor markers and the complexity of cancer biology, multiple/composite biomarkers are increasingly relied on to assess the safety and efficacy of novel anticancer drugs. The global analysis of cellular proteins has recently been termed proteomics/proteome profiling, and is a key area of research that is developing in the 'post-genome era'.

This involves the simultaneous separation, identification, and characterization of thousands of proteins present in a biological sample in a single procedure. Proteins are the main functional output, and neither the genomic DNA code of an organism nor the amount of mRNA that is expressed for each gene product yields an accurate picture on the state of a living cell, which can be altered by many conditions. In particular, post-translational modifications of proteins, such as phosphorylation or glycosylation, are very important in determining protein function (Figure 18.1).

With the use of proteomics, a whole range of protein markers can be assessed at the same time.

- Two-dimensional polyacrylamide gel electrophoresis (2D-PAGE) followed by mass spectrometry is a core technique for separating proteins on the basis of charge in one dimension and molecular mass in another. Changes in the expression of proteins can be identified by comparing the protein spots by computer-assisted photometric evaluation. This technique allows direct comparison of protein expression and is used to identify proteins that are differently expressed between normal or malignant tissue or during the course of therapy. It has also been shown to allow the detection of proteins that may be involved in the generation of resistance mechanisms.
- Surface-enhanced laser desorption ionization time-of-flight (SELD–TOF) mass spectrometry is a tool for the rapid identification of cancer-specific biomarkers and proteomic patterns in tissues or body fluids. The advantage of this technique is the high-throughput proteomic fingerprinting of samples by on-chip protein fractionation in a short period of time.

Conclusions

The evaluation of biomarkers within clinical trials is a tool to identify subgroups of patients with a high chance of responding to targeted therapy. Biomarkers allow a drug to be followed until it reaches its target and its potential effects at the tumor site to be defined. Relevant markers such as functional imaging or protein profiling may differ among the various types of targeted therapy, and are under continuous development. Much additional effort is required to define and validate novel biomarkers and develop them to surrogate markers that may add to or replace the clinical endpoints that are currently employed.

Further reading

Banks RE, Dunn MJ, Hochstrasser DF, et al. Proteomics: new perspectives, new biomedical opportunities. Lancet 2000; 18: 1749–56.

Jayson G, Jackson A, Mulatero C, et al. Molecular and biological evaluation of HuMV833 anti-VEGF antibody: resistance mechanisms in anti-angiogenic therapy. J Natl Cancer Inst 2002; 94: 1484–93.

Pao W, Miller V, Zakowski M, et al. EGF receptor gene mutations are common in lung cancers from 'never smokers' and are associated with sensitivity of tumors to gefitinib and erlotinib. Proc Natl Acad Sci USA 2004; 101: 13306–11.

Skvortsov S, Sarg B, Loeffler-Ragg J, et al. Different proteome pattern of EGFR positive colorectal cancer cell lines responsive and non-responsive to C225 antibody treatment. Mol Cancer Therapeutics 2004; 3: 1–8.

Wulfkuhle JD, Liotta LA, Petricoin EF. Proteomic applications for the early detection of cancer. Nat Rev Cancer 2003; 3: 267–75.

Index

Page numbers in *italics* refer to figures and tables